about the author

Paramananda was born John Wilson in North London in 1955. He was always curious about Eastern ideas, but it was not until the age of 23, after the death of his father, that his interest in Buddhism was aroused. The focus of his life shifted from the world of politics, in which he had been active, to more alternative ways of promoting individual and social change.

During his twenties Paramananda worked mostly as a psychiatric social worker. He has also been involved in various types of voluntary work, including the Samaritans, drug detox, and in a hospice.

In 1983 he came into contact with the Friends of the Western Buddhist Order and two years later was ordained into the Order itself. Since then he has been teaching meditation and Buddhism full-time. He sees meditation and Buddhism as powerful tools for both individual and social change, and believes that service to the community is a vital aspect of spiritual practice. He now lives in West London where he continues with his teaching and writing.

Dedicated to
Urgyen Sangharakshita
my teacher

the art of meditation

the body

paramananda

Windhorse Publications

Also by Paramananda
Change Your Mind
A Deeper Beauty

Published by
Windhorse Publications Ltd
11 Park Road
Birmingham
B13 8AB
UK
email: info@windhorsepublications.com
web: www.windhorsepublications.com

Every effort has been made to obtain permission to reprint passages
from Ryokan, *One Robe, One Bowl*, and Gwendolyn Bays (trans.),
The Voice of the Buddha (Lalitavistara). If any omission has been made
please let us know so that this may be rectified in a future edition.

Cover design: Satyadarshin
Printed by Cromwell Press Ltd, Trowbridge, England

British Library Cataloguing in Publication Data:
A catalogue record for this book is available from the British Library

ISBN: 978 1 899579 77 8

contents

introduction

I first become seriously interested in Buddhism and meditation when I was working as a counsellor in the field of mental health. I found myself increasingly frustrated in my work, as I had a growing sense that 'talking' with people was of limited use. Perhaps I was just not very good at it, but it seemed to me that there were fundamental areas of mental health left unaddressed in this method of working. Through my own practice of t'ai chi ch'uan I became convinced that working with the body on an energy level had an important role to play in promoting well-being. When this led me to meditation, I felt I had come across a practice that addressed individuals in their entirety. That was over twenty-five years ago, and since then I have been both a meditator and a meditation teacher, and I have found that meditation can be a great help to many people. While I now think that it sometimes helps to use therapies such as counselling as well, meditation offers us something of great benefit in our desire to live an authentic and happy life.

My own practice of meditation has increasingly emphasized awareness of my body, and, I feel, has become both simpler, less psychological, and more based in sensational and emotional experience as opposed to 'mental' experience. Of course, this division between mental and bodily experience is not really valid, but it does express an approach to meditation that I hope will be useful.

In a book of this size it is not possible to cover the subject as fully as I would like. Instead, my aim is to suggest ways of approaching meditation that I hope will support your own exploration. This is not, then, a manual, because meditation is not predominately a matter of technical expertise, but more akin to an art which can be mastered only through practice. So I hope this book will act as an invitation and encouragement for your own exploration of meditation. I don't wish to tell you how to meditate. Meditation cannot really *be* taught, as it is essentially a way of being with ourselves and our experience which reveals what is both universal and unique in us.

1

why the body matters

The commonest misunderstanding about meditation is that it is concerned exclusively with the mind, that it is something that we do in, and with, our heads. To use the jargon of the sixties, when meditation first became popular in the west, it is thought of as a 'head trip', an escape into a different, and perhaps higher, reality. Meditation has been associated with the counter-culture, with the orient, and with an other-worldly attitude. This is a fundamental misunderstanding. It is not an escape from the world, but a way of being more fully in the world, of becoming both more embodied, and more embedded, in the world. What do I mean by this? We will be exploring both these ideas, but perhaps a preliminary definition of these terms would be useful.

embodying
The American stand-up comedian Bill Hicks, famed for his raw honesty, had a manic and explosive routine where he railed against the mediocrity of much modern music, particularly boy bands. He cried that

he wanted his kids listening to music that came from the heart, though he put it a lot stronger than that. This is typical of Hicks, whose death at an early age robbed the world of a comedian who was prepared to say the unspeakable and make us a little more aware of the compromises and hypocrisy of modern life. Hicks' comic material is all about challenging us to be more 'real', to see what is going on around us, and to take responsibility for our lives. He considered the modern world to be 'asleep' and unwilling or unable to wake up, living a kind of half life filled with television and consumption. Like the Buddha, Hicks wanted people to wake up to what was there in front, and inside, of them, be it their lack of real connection with their children or the hypocritical foreign policy of the governments they elect. He urged people in the most forceful, and often hilarious, manner, to reconnect with themselves in their full richness and depth. He wanted rock singers who sang from their 'fucking hearts'. We might not all relate to his raw style, but many of us will be sympathetic to his call. Hicks' comedy was embodied, in that it came from his heart; deeply felt and forcefully expressed. When something comes from the heart it has a power to it, a quality that marks it out. That power does not have to be angry or raw; it might also be subtle and gentle, as with this poem by the Buddhist hermit monk Ryokan, written in the eighteenth century.

> The night is fresh and cool –
> Staff in hand, I walk through the gate.
> Wisteria and ivy grow together along the winding
>   mountain path;

*Birds sing quietly in their nests and a monkey
    howls nearby.*
*As I reach a high peak a village appears in the
    distance.*
The old pines are full of poems;
I bend down for a drink of pure spring water.
*There is a gentle breeze, and the round moon hangs
    overhead.*
Standing by a deserted building,
*I pretend to be a crane softly floating among the
    clouds.*[1]

I come at this idea of embodiment through comedy
and poetry because, like these art forms, it cannot
really be neatly pinned down. Embodiment is a quality of being that expresses a connection to the feeling
side of us, to both the heart and the guts of us. It is no
coincidence that we use words like 'heart' and 'guts'
to try to express a quality of authenticity and depth.
They are more than metaphors. They capture the
experiential quality of being embodied. We feel in our
bodies. When we are disconnected from the blood
and bones of ourselves, we are lost to ourselves. To be
embodied means to 'be at home', to be present and
alive to our felt experience.

For me, this is what meditation is concerned with
above all: a coming home to our hearts, a coming
home to what the poet David White calls 'the house of
belonging'.

embedding
I recently watched a television programme about the
culture of the indigenous people of Australia. I was

struck by their intimacy with the world around them. I was impressed not only by their vast knowledge of plants and animals, but also by their sense of care and appreciation for their environment, a profound sense of belonging within the landscape that brought forth a feeling of reverence and responsibility for the world that sustained them. They seemed totally at home in the world, in a deep, yet relaxed, intimacy with everything around them. Of course, it is easy to project on to people who appear to live in a more connected and authentic manner than oneself, but there is little doubt that many of us have lost a sense of belonging in the world. The challenge that faces us, individually and collectively, is to find a way of being in the world that respects that world and offers us a real feeling of belonging and involvement. So when I use the term 'embedded', this is the kind of thing I am trying to express: a sense of care, connection, and belonging, towards both the world itself and those with whom we share it. I believe this sense of embeddedness springs from being embodied. When we are more fundamentally connected to ourselves, we also become more connected to the world around us, for if we are not comfortable in our own skins, how can we hope to feel at ease in the world?

the role of the body
The body is critical to these ideas of embodiment and embeddedness, for it is in and through the body that we feel our connection with our deeper selves and the world around us. I am not suggesting that thinking is unimportant – the right kind of thinking is vital – but I do want to suggest there is something more

primal about feeling, that thinking comes after feeling, in both our collective and our individual evolution, and that losing touch with this embodied sense of ourselves, based in sensation and emotion, is to lose the ground of our being and leave our thoughts abstracted from ourselves and our surroundings. When we become disconnected in this way, we lose contact with the feeling bodies that ground us, and find ourselves dominated by our egos, with the world shrunk to the size of our heads. We are plagued with anxiety and self-referential worries. The world is just a backdrop to the drama that is us. This is now such a common state of mind that we think it is normal, but Buddhist meditation suggests that a very different state is not only possible but far more enjoyable, and characterized by awareness and compassion. In this process of moving away from self-obsession and worry towards openness and compassion it is vital to fundamentally reconnect with ourselves, and this means reawakening the body as an instrument of feeling, sensation, and aliveness.

I hope that gives you some sense of what I am trying to get at by employing these terms. I do want to stress that they are not meant technically; they are meant poetically – that is, they are to be explored in relation to your experience and felt into. Here, then, is a meditation to start to get a feel for being embodied.

a few general notes about meditation
Before you try this meditation, I want to make a few general remarks about all the meditations in this book. First, if you are not used to meditation you

might wish to read the next chapter, on posture, before you start.

Try to approach meditation with a sense of curiosity and kindness towards yourself. As long as you are aware of your experience, you cannot do it wrong. Just be interested in what your experience really is, rather than having a idea of what it should be like. Try to foster a non-judgemental attitude. Feel free to stop at any point if that feels appropriate. Try not to force anything. If you get really uncomfortable, don't sit there in pain, move carefully, but try not to fidget. Make sure you have plenty of time, and don't rush anything.

After the meditation, take a few minutes to reflect on your experience. Some people find it useful to take a few notes as an aid to reflection.

Read through the meditation a couple of times and then try it for yourself. Don't worry about following the instructions to the letter, just try to have a sense of the practice, and see what happens.

meditation: awareness and the body

> *Sit in your chosen meditation posture with your eyes closed. Become aware of your face; just notice what it feels like. Notice how sensitive the skin of your face is, the feel of the air against the skin. Imagine your face softening a little, particularly the brow, around your eyes, and your jaw. You might try linking this to your breath, by imagining your face relaxing especially on your out-breath. If you use your breath in this way, just breathe naturally; don't try to control it. Try not to*

form a judgement about how your face feels. Notice if you are thinking, 'oh, my jaw is really clenched,' and then let go of those thoughts. Take your time.

Become aware of your scalp, and notice any sensations on the crown of your head. You may wish to recall what is above your head – above your room: the sky. Imagine your scalp softening a little against the roundness of your skull. Let your awareness move down the back of your head to the base of your skull. See if you can have a sense of where the skull and the spine meet. This is quite high up, about level with the ears, and quite deep set, almost in the centre of the head. You might try slightly nodding your head backwards and forwards from this point. Imagine the muscles at the base of your head softening a little, encouraging the idea that you do not have to hold on to your head, it will just balance there on top of your spine.

Now begin to let a sense of awareness spread down across your shoulders. If they feel tight or held, you might like to imagine your awareness as a warm golden light encouraging your shoulders to relax.

Allow your awareness to spread across and down your back, just giving your back some attention. Imagine your back being broad and long. Notice any feeling or sensations behind your heart.

If your thoughts drift, don't worry, just bring them gently back when you notice. If any images or thoughts arise that relate to being aware of your body, you might want to just dwell on them for a few moments. For instance, when you become aware of the area behind your heart, a thought or an image might come to mind.

Don't try to make this sort of thing happen, but if it does, spend a few moments with it.

After taking in your back, let the awareness gather at the base of your spine, then imagine your spine gently curving up through your body. Imagine the spine as it is, full of life, made up of connective tissues as well as bones. Bring your awareness back to the base of your spine, and then let it spread through the pelvic area, taking in the shape of your pelvis and including your genitals.

Now begin to notice all the sensations that arise from your contact with your seat or your cushion and the floor. Try to let go of your buttocks and legs, imagine completely surrendering the lower body to gravity. Feel the weight of the big bones in your thighs, and the large muscles, and give their weight to the ground. Be aware of the ground fully supporting you. Let go with the out-breath as completely as you are able. It helps to remember the earth beneath you unconditionally. Let yourself become aware of your legs, imagine releasing into the hips, knees, and ankles, even the small joints of your feet. In your imagination, encourage the soles of your feet to soften.

Now bring your awareness to the lowest point in your body at which you feel it responding to your breath. This will probably be below your navel. Use your breathing to support awareness of your body. Become more aware of your body on the in-breath, and cultivate a sense of letting go on the out-breath.

Notice any feelings or thoughts connected with being aware of your belly, then move your awareness slowly

*up the front of your body, taking in the ribcage, and
how it opens to receive your breath. Breathe awareness
into your body. Be aware of the heart and the upper
chest area. Then move your awareness down your arms
and into your hands. Gather your awareness in your
hands for a few moments, noticing the sensations in the
palms and fingers. Then just sit for a while being aware
of your body breathing.*

Don't feel you have to stick slavishly to these instructions. You might feel inclined to spend more time on
some areas of your body rather than others, but make
sure you include your whole body. Some places
might feel a little numb or dull, and you find hard it to
be aware of them. Just notice if this is the case; don't
try to force your awareness into those areas. It is very
important that you approach the whole exercise with
a sense of kindness and being open to your experience. Don't have unrealistic expectations. In all likelihood your mind will wander. This doesn't mean you
are doing anything wrong; it is the same for
everyone.

drawing your body
As an aid to body awareness, you might try drawing a
picture of your body after a meditation such as the
one described above. Rather than draw an accurate
representation of your body, use colour and shape to
give an emotional, impressionistic image. Forget
about it looking like you, or even having a human
shape. Don't even think about it, just start drawing
and see what comes. You might use colour to express
the feelings when you brought awareness to the different areas of your body. If drawing is not your

thing, an alternative is to write about your experience, but again let go of any ideas about good writing and see what comes out when you don't think about it too much.

the body and the mind

I have suggested there are misunderstandings about meditation. There are many types of meditation, but I am talking about the Buddhist understanding of meditation and my experience of meditating within that tradition. I have already suggested that many people think meditation is about what goes on in our heads. One reason for this is the western understanding of 'mind' as opposed to the eastern one. There is also the western emphasis on the centrality of rationality as the defining characteristic of the human being, and the resulting dualistic view of the mind and body. It is easy to get caught up in words such as 'mind' and 'awareness'. I often notice this when I teach meditation. People want to understand what all these different terms mean, but to really understand the mind you need to study it, not abstractly or theoretically but through noticing what is happening in our own minds. When we do this we begin to 'feel' that the division between mind and body has no experiential validity. Perhaps this is because meditation, which is a great way of noticing what is going on in our own minds, has been an important part of eastern cultures for thousands of years, that oriental people tend not to split the mind and the body in the way western people do. Whatever the reasons, the eastern idea of mind very much includes all aspects of our experience, not just our conscious thoughts, so when it comes to working with the mind in meditation, this is also understood to involve the whole of the human being.

So meditation is just as concerned with the body as with the mind, or – more correctly – it is concerned with all aspects of us. Meditation is, then, a way of working with the body-mind complex that makes us who and what we are. One of the principal benefits of meditation is that it brings us into a fuller relationship with the various aspects of ourselves which tend to become separated in our everyday experience of ourselves. This separation is reflected by the way we talk. When we say that someone is in their head, or all heart, or heartless, or hard-headed, this suggests a tendency for aspects of ourselves to become split from one another. In western culture there is also a tendency to live on a predominately mental level, where the sensational and feeling side of our experience becomes increasingly less available to us, at least on a moment-to-moment basis. For example, when you walk down the street how aware are you of your body, your feet on the earth, the sky above you? Do you really notice the world around you? During our everyday activities, many of us are barely aware of our bodies or the world around us, being caught up in the endless chatter in our heads.

Take a moment now just to notice how you are sitting as you read these words. Take a couple of slightly deeper breaths and see if you can relax any tensions you become aware of. It is very useful to get into the habit of noticing your body now and then, coming back to the physical side of your experience from time to time throughout the day. It can be as simple as taking three conscious breaths and relaxing your face and shoulders. Tension in the body builds up gradually through the days and years. Getting into the practice of just noticing your body a little more can be a great help in reducing such tension.

I now want to say a little about why the body is so vital to meditation. Most people's experience of themselves and the world soon after they are born is predominately physical: we know we are hungry because we feel hunger, and we express this very directly thorough crying. There is no thought involved, not in the way we normally speak of it. Our experience of being in the world is very direct, physical, and immediate. As we grow, we learn to communicate, and our expression and experience becomes increasingly subject to thought. This, of course, is how it should be, but it seems that this process often goes too far, and may be made worst by unfortunate experiences when we are young, until we eventually lose the spontaneous qualities that are so evident in healthy young children. For instance, when did you last jump for joy? This is something that small children do daily. It is as if the experience and expression of ourselves through our bodies becomes buried under all the mental chatter in our heads. I am not suggesting that it is in any way wrong to be thoughtful about our lives, but that it is possible to be both thoughtful and grown up, and still be in touch with the physical joy of being alive, and that it is possible to be moved to tears by a beautiful sunset and still be a mature and rational adult.

What tends to happen as we grow older is that felt experiences – the feelings and emotions that happen within, and are naturally expressed through, the body – become increasing unavailable to us, and we feel somewhat numb and alienated from ourselves. I am not going to delve into why this happens, it is enough to note that there are many theories. It is, however, worth noting that there seems to be a relationship between our ability to experience and express emotion through the body and our mental well-being. Put simply, if we hold everything inside we become unhappy. One of the reasons people come to meditation classes is that they feel cut off from some aspects of themselves, and intuitively wish to regain the aliveness they once felt.

Although at first sight it might seem that meditation is largely a mental process, this is not really the case. Meditation is about becoming, or perhaps I should say rebecoming. It is about rediscovering ourselves. It offers us a chance to be intimate with ourselves, to re-claim aspects of ourselves that have been lost. This is of course just one way of talking about meditation, and I hope one of the things that will become clear is that meditation is a very rich and deep activity that can be experienced and discussed in many ways. In this book, we will focus on the physical aspects of this profound practice.

what do we mean by the mind?
As I have already said, the idea of mind, in the East in general and in Buddhism in particular, is rather different from the one we usually have in the West. Although it is used in many different ways in western

culture, we normally use it to refer to our faculty for conscious thought, particularly rational thought. If we say that someone has a good mind, we mean he or she is intelligent and thinks clearly. On the other hand, if we say that someone acted mindlessly, we mean he or she acted without thinking things through, without considering the consequences. We also speak sometimes as though there is a split between mind and heart, and between mind and body. We tend to think of mind as something that can be separated from feelings and emotions.

This is very different from the idea of mind found in Buddhism. Buddhism's idea of mind, and in particular mindfulness, very much includes our feelings, on the level of physical sensations and emotions. I will say more about this later, but for now I want to make it clear that the concept of mind I will be using includes bodily sensations and emotions. Meditation, then, is concerned with working with all aspects of our minds, for, according to the Buddhist tradition, physical feelings and emotions are a very important part of how we experience ourselves, and meditation is primarily about our day-to-day, even moment-to-moment, experience of ourselves.

Meditation aims to help us become increasingly aware of ourselves in the moment. Awareness is really the key to meditation, both in the sense that it is what we are, above all, trying to develop through meditation, and also in the sense that it is the quality of mind that allows us to meditate in the first place. Awareness really means simply being alive to our experience. It means that we know what we are doing in a very basic sense. We know what we are doing with our bodies, that is, our posture and our movements, what we are feeling – whether we happy or sad – and what we are thinking: the quality and content of our thoughts at any given time. This all sounds very basic, and it is. Meditation is a very simple sort of activity. We might have the idea that meditation is about a very special kind of experience, i.e. spiritual experience, and although this is one aspect of meditation, it is not really the most important, which is to be aware of what is really happening is a down-to-earth, simple and direct way.

A traditional Buddhist story[2] tells how a king once asked a renowned teacher to tell him the most profound teaching of the Buddha. He wanted to know the higher teachings, the teachings that would lead him to Enlightenment. The teacher simply said to the king, 'Attention.' The king was disappointed with this and questioned the teacher further, demanding the full teachings, to which the teacher replied, 'Attention, attention, attention!' In other words, the most important thing is to pay attention to what is happening in the moment. There are quite a lot of these stories within Buddhism, they are designed to impress on us the fact that Buddhist practice, particularly meditation, is really very simply: it involves paying careful and kind attention to whatever is really happening.

I hope you are not also disappointed with this answer. Sometimes it is easy to believe there is an answer out there that will make sense of our lives, something we can find out that will make everything right, but that is just a fantasy. There is no teaching out there that is going to put everything right, and instantly make us wise and content. If we want to change, we have to start with our experience as it is now, make a consistent effort, and be prepared for this process to take a long time. This is not as bad as it might sound, for when it comes to using meditation as a way to change ourselves, the process itself is both valuable and enjoyable, at least most of the time. Many meditators find that they can't imagine their lives without it, become less and less concerned with whatever goal they started out with, and find themselves more content and happy with how they are on a day-to-day basis. And this really is the point of meditation; it helps us to get the most out of our lives, to enjoy ourselves, and to appreciate others and the world around us. People who have been meditating for a while sometimes realize they have spent their lives wanting to achieve something, or wanting to be different, and in all that wanting they have forgotten to enjoy life as it is and appreciate the good things they already have.

The quality of mind that allows us to do that, to take in and enjoy what is there in front of us, inside us, is known as 'mindfulness', and this is at the heart of the Buddha's teaching and at the core of meditation.

Mindfulness is a particular quality of mind. It is sometimes equated with concentration, but this can be misleading. Concentration reminds me of being trapped in school when all I wanted was to be out in the sunshine, and our teacher demanding that we concentrate on what he thought we should be doing.

This experience of associating concentration with forcing oneself to pay attention is fairly common. Although mindfulness can rightly be said to have a strong element of concentration, this is of a particular type. It is not forced, and it has the feeling of being pleasurable. It is perhaps better spoken of as absorption or engagement, the kind of feeling you have when you are really enjoying yourself.

Bring to mind an activity that you like. It could be as everyday as reading a good book. When you are doing that, your mind is full of what you are doing, and not doing anything else, such as wishing you were somewhere else, or caught up in thinking about the future. This is closer to the sort of mindfulness that we look for during meditation. There is no sense of having to force the mind. It is engaged and content to be employed in what it is doing. In meditation, the mind is turned towards one's moment-to-moment experience. As we shall see later, in more detail, part of this experience is that of having a body. It is through this awareness of the body that one comes more fully into oneself, in terms of feelings and emotions. We are no longer caught in the continuous chatter of the mind, but there is a sense of fullness, of wholeness, based on being in touch with one's living, breathing body.

thinking is not the same as awareness
The principal function of the brain is to map, monitor, and manage the body of which it is a part, and regulate the internal environment of the body in relationship to the external environment, of which it is also a part. That is to say, it is aware of the sensations and

feelings, and utilizes the sense information in relation to the world around it. Clearly, the mind of a human being has evolved to do rather more than this basic brain. It has developed the ability to think self-consciously. This remarkable development means that we can make choices about how we respond to an enormous variety of situations. Although we take this self-reflective awareness for granted, it is a truly mysterious faculty. One of the consequences is that we have a sense of selfhood, we feel there is something in there making our decisions. We are also aware that this 'something' experiences a wide range of emotions, from delight to despair and everything in between. Because this is what it feels like, it becomes very hard not to feel that this something is separate from everything else and needs promoting and protecting. It is, then, a strange paradox that this self-reflective awareness, which so remarkably allows us to be aware of ourselves and the world around us, also creates a sense of separation, from ourselves, other people, and the world. We experience our bodies, other people, and the world as objects, with ourselves as the subject. Our response to this strange situation is central to the teachings of Buddhism. How should we deal with this remarkable gift of self-reflective awareness? One possibility is to be selfish, to try to sustain this delusion of a separate fixed self in whatever way we can. It is this selfishness that gives rise to craving, for craving is the desire to satisfy this feeling we have of being a separate self.

Buddhism is deeply disturbing to this feeling of selfhood, for it asks us to realize that selfhood is a delusion created by our self-reflective awareness. Furthermore, it tells us that it is by strengthening the very thing that has created the delusion that we can see through it. This is not a easy thing to grasp. We might understand it on an intellectual level, but we continue to behave as a self, distinct and separate from everything else.

It is very hard to think ourselves out of the idea of such a self, because our ability to think, the ability to abstract from direct experience, feels as though it is dependent on the abstraction of an idea of a self. It is our faculty for abstract thought that creates the abstraction of a self. The Buddhist teaching of 'no self' has led to a lot of confusion. It is quite hard to explain, and it has often led to the idea, at least in the West, that the ego or self should be destroyed. For most people, this sort of approach is unhelpful. It is a macho and paradoxical egocentric approach that goes against the spirit of love and kindness so central to Buddhism, whose solution to this problem is mindfulness. Mindfulness is not about killing off the ego, but more of an opening up of our sense of self to include other people and the world. It is an opening up to the richness and complexity of our own being, for our ego tries to confine us, restricts our experience to what it believes supports its own existence, like a miser obsessed with his meagre treasure when all around is beauty and richness. But the ego is really very insecure, and easily threatened. It has to be gradually coaxed to relax its grip on our experience. Rather like a dog that has been ill treated, it needs kindness and even a bit of humour; it won't respond positively to bullying.

There are, of course, other approaches, and for a full-time monk or nun under the guidance of a skilled master these might be effective, but this is not the case for most of us. When we read about a Zen monk gaining insight on being struck by the master's staff, we have to take into account the context and the relationship between the master and the student.

When Buddhism refers to awareness and mindfulness, it is concerned with strengthening and extending the self-reflective aspect of the mind. Mindfulness is concerned with the application of this special quality of the human mind to be aware of itself, and aware of direct experience. This kind of awareness is not the same as thought. Imagine being in a beautiful place. Our awareness of that beauty is something we feel – we do not 'think' beauty. Once we think how beautiful a landscape is, we start to lose contact with the actual sense of beauty; the words and thoughts get in the way of the experience. It is the same with many other things: our thoughts lead us away from direct awareness of what is happening. I remember how I used to be very aware of this when I worked in a hospice. I sat with people who were close to death, and I noticed how I would often start thinking and lose awareness of the situation. My practice was one of trying just to be with the dying person as fully as possible. I found it most useful to stay with a sense of my own body, my own breath, to try to remain embodied, and then I was more able to be there with that person.

The mind is not just a thinking machine; it also allows us to be aware of our bodily sensations and emotional states and thoughts. The brain is not just the grey matter inside your skull, but is better understood as a complex system spread throughout our bodies which includes all our senses. We can think of the mind as this system plus the special quality of self-reflective awareness. (This is not exclusively a human thing, recent research with other primates has clearly shown that they also have the ability for such emotions as empathy, emotions that would not be possible without some degree of self-reflective awareness.) This ability to be aware is not the same as thinking, it is more of a feeling. We do not think em-pathy; we feel it. So mindfulness is about being aware of these feelings, as well as our thoughts.

To get an idea of what I mean, try becoming aware of your hands, and recall all the different tasks that you do with your hands – everyday things like washing, dressing, preparing breakfast. See if you can feel one of those tasks in your hands. It is as though your hands know what to do; you don't have to tell them how to perform these tasks, some of which are very delicate and require sensitivity. Our hands have awareness within them – as does the body in general. The vast majority of tasks don't require much think-ing; we would be in trouble if they did. I am reminded of this sort of body learning when I practise t'ai chi ch'uan. The form I learned over twenty years ago is now in my body, that is to say, my body knows how to do it. What I find interesting about this is that if I think about it, I can't do it. If I think what movement comes next, I invariably get it wrong, the pattern of movement breaks up. Nevertheless, when I am doing it I am very aware of what I am doing. I am aware how my body feels, how it is moving, the shifting of weight, the sensations of energy, and so on. So there can be awareness without thinking. Mindfulness is this kind of awareness: it is a knowing that is not thought but directly felt. Although this might sound a little strange, mindfulness can also be applied to thoughts themselves. We can be aware of our thoughts without adding to the thinking, and then we notice the feeling of thought more than the actual content.

Suppose you are meditating and you become aware that you are thinking about work. Maybe you have some problem at work. Try to be aware of the texture or feeling of those thoughts. Are they anxious, or perhaps angry? If they have an emotional texture, can you feel any related sensations in your body? Perhaps you have tightened up in your belly or in your face. Perhaps there is a feeling of energy or heat. In this way, we are trying to reunite our thoughts with our feeling aspect, there is a 're-membering' of thought to the body and the heart.

Mindfulness is a quality of awareness that does not require us to think. Consequently it does not involve the maintenance of the delusion of a self. We are aware, but we do not add to this awareness the idea of a self that is aware. In this way, it is a kind of awareness that is embodied; we acquire a sense of the mind as part of us rather than as something separate. Mindfulness, then, is the beginning of loosening our self's hold on our experience. It offers the possibility of being aware of our direct experience without adding the abstraction of selfhood. The foundation of this mindfulness is discovered by directing our awareness towards our direct experience of our bodies in terms of sensation, feelings, and emotions.

There is one exercise I have found very useful in working with thoughts, particularly the kind of thoughts that seem to arise from the ego's attempts to impose itself on our direct experience. According to the Tibetan tradition, our ego is seated in the lower abdomen. This way of thinking comes from looking at ourselves in terms of energy, and is related to the idea of chakras, or energy centres. In this exercise we use our breath to become more aware of the lower abdomen, and encourage our breathing to become a little deeper than usual. For this particular version, I am indebted to the Buddhist writer and teacher Dr Reginald Ray.

abdominal breathing

Wearing non-restrictive clothing, lie on the floor on a thin mat or blanket, and make sure you are warm and comfortable. I find it helpful to rest my head on a book so that my neck is free, the book under the base of my skull elevating my head a little so that it is aligned with my spine. Just lie there for a while, letting the ground fully support your body. Cultivate a sense of the whole earth beneath you, supporting you.

When your body has settled, become aware of your breath. At first, just notice it, feel it in your body, sustaining you. Now take a slightly deeper in-breath so that you feel you are using the whole of your lungs, with a sense of the in-breath going right down to the belly.

As you breath in, gently roll the hips away from you so that your back is slightly arched. As you breath out, roll your hips towards you so that you are pushing the small of your back towards the floor. Practise this gentle rolling of the hips for a few breaths until you have a feel for how it allows the breath to deepen. Over the course of the next twelve breaths you are going to strengthen the exhalations, keeping the in-breath the same, just a little stronger than your natural breath, and gradually try to push out more and more air on the out-breath by using the muscles of the pelvic floor and then the lower abdomen. These are the muscles you use when you interrupt urination. Women who have had babies will know about these from their prenatal classes.

To begin with, gently tighten the muscles of your pelvic floor and then the lower abdomen in order to push out the air, still rolling your hips as you breathe. Then use your diaphragm to push out all the air. As you go through the cycle of twelve breaths, increase the effort so that by about ten breaths you are making a real effort to push out all the air. Don't overdo it, but make as much effort as you can without straining yourself. After the twelfth out-breath just relax.

Repeat the whole cycle twice more, relaxing for a few minutes between each cycle. When you have completed three cycles of abdominal breathing, just breathe naturally again, becoming aware what your body feels like.

You might feel a sense of energy and vitality in the body, a sense of the body having been invigorated.

Once you have got used to this exercise, you can also try it sitting in meditation posture. I have found that this simple exercise really helps people to be more aware of their bodies when they meditate, and it is a very useful exercise to make part of your meditation practice. There seems to be a direct relationship between distraction and the failure to fully exhale all the breath from the body. It is as if the stale air in the body encourages the mind to be dull and distracted, whereas fully exhaling clears the mind and strengthens the awareness. So in addition to doing the abdominal breathing before you start meditation, if you find yourself distracted by stale thoughts you might try emphasizing your out-breath and make sure that you exhale fully.

2

posture

When people consider the role of the body in meditation, they often do so in relation to posture. When we think about posture we often see it as a bit of a problem. We like the idea of a perfect posture, to be able to sit still and upright without difficulty or pain. If we have a 'good' posture we might even be proud of it and look down our noses at people who shuffle around in the meditation room. For the rest of us, the body often seems to get in the way of meditation. 'If only I felt comfortable I would be able to meditate,' 'If only my bum wasn't so numb,' and so on. The first thing I want to emphasize is that bodily posture is not something extra to meditation to be tolerated or corrected. The body and its posture is meditation. I often say this sort of thing to students these days. I will say meditate with your body, not with your head, or that meditation happens in the body, not in the head. Of course, the dualism is false, but I am trying to get across the point that the body is vital to meditation, and to think of meditation as something that happens in the head is misguided.

This is made very clear if we take a look at the *Satipatthana Sutta*, which is one of the most important, if not *the* most important, Buddhist texts on meditation. The text gives detailed and comprehensive instructions on the practice of mindfulness for the attainment of insight. According to the sutta, the first concern for our awareness is the body. The advice given on posture is as follows.

> *Here, O bhikkhus, a bhikkhu, gone to the forest, to the foot of a tree, or to an empty place, sits down, bends in his legs crosswise on his lap, keeps his body erect, and arouses mindfulness in the object of meditation, namely, the breath which is in front of him.*[3]

Although the sutta goes on to give detailed instruction concerning awareness of the body, it does not tell us very much about posture. This might be because people in India were used to sitting on the ground, and their posture had not been subject to the distorting influence of modern furniture. Most of us will not be able to achieve the 'full lotus' position referred to, but the general principle is clear: we are looking for a stable, grounded basis and an upright torso. (I am not very happy with the term 'erect', as it sounds a little stiff.) We will now look at three related aspects of posture: alignment, relaxation, and aliveness.[4]

alignment
the pelvis
I am lucky enough to have a three-year old son. A while ago I bought him some old-fashioned wooden bricks, which I can remember from my own childhood. I often find myself sitting on the floor with him

making towers. It is possible to build quite a high tower if the bricks are aligned carefully. If they are not stacked just right, they soon become unstable and topple over. Although the parts of our bodies are all connected, the basic principle of alignment still applies. Gravity exerts a constant downward force on us, so if we are well aligned, it becomes a supportive force and provides stability. If our bodies are not aligned, it will take a good deal of muscular effort to resist the force of gravity.

When we are sitting, our torso balances from the pelvis, so the pelvis is one of the key areas for our attention. Our ability to sit upright is determined largely by our positioning the pelvis at the correct angle. It is very important to make sure that, however you sit, the pelvis is always higher than the knees. Just how far above the knees will vary from one person to another, but your knees should never be higher than your pelvis, even when you are sitting on a chair. It is important to pay close attention to how your posture feels. Even though both our posture and awareness of our bodies might have become distorted through years of misuse, we can, with careful, kindly attention, learn what the body intuitively knows.

Something else I have learned from my son, just by watching him, is how naturally balanced children's bodies are. If you want to know how to sit on the floor with ease, take a look at a three-year-old. As adults, most of us have to pay a bit more attention to our bodies if we want to be comfortable. Incidentally, the word 'comfortable' is an interesting term; 'fort' is related to strength, while 'com' is an intensifier. So it means something like 'much strength', which is perhaps not what we think of as comfort.

But back to the pelvis. We probably don't take much notice of our pelvis unless it starts to play up. So the first thing to do is to get more of a feel for it. You might literally like to have a feel of it now. Feel your hips, sit on your hands and feel the base of the pelvis. Get up and move it around a little. Think of Elvis – a man who knew where his pelvis was! Enjoy having a pelvis. We need to get a sense of the shape of our pelvis. If you are not sure, have a look at *Gray's Anatomy*. Try to develop a feeling for how your pelvis connects with your spine. Notice what it feels like to bring a little awareness to this area of your body.

Let's have another go at sitting on our hands, I know it sounds odd, but it is a really good way of getting a feel for the angle of your pelvis when you sit, and this is a vital factor in allowing the body to move into its natural alignment. Using some cushions or a chair, sit on your hands with your palms up. You should be able to feel part of your pelvis. Rock gently backwards and forwards on your hands. The bone you feel should become more or less prominent as you rock. That bone feels most prominent when the pelvis is upright. Slowly rock less and less until you come to a stop. Now do the same thing again, but this time without your hands underneath you. You might find you have to adjust the height of your cushions in order to sit comfortably with your pelvis upright. The height of the cushions influences the angle of your pelvis, and if you are too low you will need to add another cushion. If you are too high, you will need to take a cushion away. This height adjustment is important, and the degree of adjustment can be quite fine, so if possible keep a variety of cushions to experiment with. Firm cushions are best. If you do not have proper meditation cushions, try rolling up a pillow. I have found this to work well.

the head
The other main area of the body that you need to be aware of, in relation to this idea of getting the body aligned, is the head. Now heads are rather heavy, some heads are heavier than others, and if they are not balanced quite a lot of effort is required to keep them up. In any case, we tend to hold a lot of tension in our necks. Many people go through life with their heads slightly pulled back, leading with the chin, and this means that the neck and the muscles at the base of the skull are somewhat compressed. In this case, you might initially find it feels odd when your head is properly balanced, or you might find it hard to know when it is balanced. If so, it's good to get someone else to have a look at you; otherwise try sitting in front of a mirror. You are looking to get your head to balance in line with your spine. This is not easy to see in a mirror, but from the front you should be able to tell if you are pulling back your head, or if it is dropped too far forward.

Again, the main thing is to try to bring some awareness to this area. Don't think you have to get it exactly right, just try to sense what is going on in your neck. I have found it useful to gain a sense of the point where the skull and spine meet. It is more or less in the middle of the head, and quite deep. With your fingers, find the hollows behind your ear lobes. This gives you the level of the top of your spine, and the point where the skull pivots on the spine is a little way in from this level, towards the back of the head. Because the greater mass of the head is forward from this pivot, the head would fall forward and down if the neck muscles were completely relaxed, so when you start to fall asleep, your head will fall forwards. Because of this gravitational pull, we tend to over-compensate and build up tension in the neck. We hold on to our heads much more than we really need to. This is a bit of a metaphor for the way many of us go about our lives, with a sense of having to hold on in case it starts to fall apart, or we lose our heads.

Ideally, there is a dynamic tension in the muscles of the back of the neck to prevent the head becoming held through too much tension, which pulls the head back and down. This tendency is very common in westerners. Have a look at people in the street and you will see this sort of thing in the majority of adults. If you look at young children you'll notice there is quite a difference.

It is rather difficult to adjust your own head, but you can bear what I have said in mind and try to imagine a sense of freedom at the pivot point I have described. It is not hard to find an Alexander Technique teacher, and it is well worth a visit to one as they will, I am sure, be able to give you an experiential sense of what I am saying. Otherwise, visit your local library, as there are plenty of books on the subject. It is particularly worth trying out the Alexander supine posture, in which you lay on your back with your head supported by a book, with the neck free, as this will give you a sense of what it feels like to have your head correctly aligned.

Many postural problems involve the position of the head. Again, this may require very subtle adjustment. Later on, I will describe a meditation that should help give you get a feeling for this. For now, try making very small movements of your head, and see if you can get a sense of where the skull meets the spine and any movement at that point. Then see if you can get a sense of the back of your neck being fully extended. Imagine your neck long and soft, and your head poised on your spine. Imagine that you don't need to hold on to your head but that it can just balance there with a minimum of dynamic tension in the your neck.

The main thing I want to emphasize about posture is that it should be an ongoing process of awareness in your meditation. We don't just get it right and then forget about it. Our posture forms the basis of our meditation and should be understood as integral to it. So rather than see your posture as a problem that stops you enjoying your meditation, see it as part of your practice, as a vital aspect of you, which you are learning to love and bring awareness to. Our attitude towards our posture, taking into consideration whatever limitations your particular body might have, is clearly connected to our overall attitude to our bodies. And as I hope will become clear, this is of central concern in relation to our meditation, indeed to our lives in general. At the same time, don't become neurotic about your posture. Try to relate to it in a spirit of inquiry. This is a good attitude to meditation in general: paying attention is a chance to find out more about yourself. You don't have to achieve an ideal posture, just learn to work with what you have in a relaxed and open way.

the arms and hands
The way you hold your arms and hands is also important. If you have upper back pain, between the shoulders or in the neck, this might be because of the position of your arms. The most common problem is that the hands are too low down. This causes the shoulders to be pulled forward and the upper back becomes rounded. If they are resting on your thighs, your hands need to be quite high up the leg, nearer to your hips than your knees. I prefer to hold them palms down, but finding the best individual posture is often a matter of trial and error. One alternative is to hold the hands a little below the navel, or rest them on an upright cushion. Or you can try wrapping a blanket round the top of your hips and tucking the hands into it just below the navel. In some forms of Zen meditation, the hands form a particular gesture – the cosmic mudra – and this works well for some people. One hand supports the other in front of the navel, palms upwards, with the thumbs gently touching. Something else I have found useful is to become aware of my elbows and to think of them falling towards the floor. This seems to help to release the shoulders, another area where tension accumulates.

the face
When I lead people through a body relaxation, I tend to spend a lot of time on the face. I am not sure why I started to do this, I just found myself talking more

and more about softening and relaxing in the face. Perhaps it is because this is where we often see tension. It is the most public area of our bodies, where we are on display to the world. We have a lot of control over our faces. We try to present a certain face to the world, and we are careful in case our facial expression gives us away. It is not only poker players who learn to control their faces.

However, it is hard to get the face to do what you want and to look natural at the same time. This is one reason why acting is a lot more difficult than it appears. It is hard make a smile convincing if the associated emotions are not there. So we might find we go through the day holding our face; we grin and bear it, as the expression goes. We might find that we hold our face not only against the outer world, but also with regard to our own emotions, though perhaps this is a particularly English trait in the form of the stiff upper lip. The English are not the only ones, of course, as I found when I lived in California, although the required expression there is a little different. People involved in retail, especially, always seem to be smiling, which their customers may find pleasant, though for someone from England it can be a little disconcerting.

So the face is a very good place to begin the process of relaxation. Think more of becoming aware of your face than forcing it to relax. Tell yourself that at least in meditation you don't have to put on a face. Zen people sometimes talk about 'finding your natural face before you were born'. As with rather a lot of Zen sayings, it's a bit hard to know what this is getting at, but I find it a useful idea. Imagining your face before it was born suggests a sense of freedom from the pressures of daily life. It's an encouragement to let go of world-weariness and relax into a space in which you are not subject to the judgement of the ego.

More pragmatically, try exploring your face with your hands. Be quite firm. Feel around the eye sockets with your fingers, feel into the hinge of the jaw and give your temples a firm rub. Try to get a sense of the shape of your skull. Move the jaw around, from side to side and up and down. Use your hands to encourage awareness in your face. Then just sit and imagine the face letting go. Don't tell your face that it must relax, just imagine it softening. Imagine your face naturally expressing how you feel as you sit there, just as you are now. See if you can let go of your jaw a little, and let the tongue rest gently on the roof of your mouth, just behind the front teeth.

I haven't said anything about the modern visual obsession with the face, the trend towards the normalization of face-lifts, botox, and the like. One of the strangest experiences of my life was a night-time bus ride from a motel on the edge of Las Vegas to the Strip. The bus was brightly lit and full of what appeared to be relatively youthful passengers. But there was something wrong, a feeling that all was not as it seemed. It was like a scene from a zombie movie. I started to notice that their faces didn't work properly, they didn't move in the way the human face is meant to move. Then I noticed that many of these faces where supported by necks that appeared some decades older. It was a bizarre trip among the eternally youthful. It is odd to contrast this with those wonderful old photographs you can find of Native Americans, their faces lined like riverbeds, and full of self-blessing.

the belly

Just below our navels is our core – at least in an energy sense. While we might experience the heart as our emotional centre, our energetic centre is lower down, below our navel. It is of course through the navel that we first received nourishment, it was here that we were connected to our mothers. This area is associated with emotion – often of the primal kind. Fear, anger, rage, as well as contentment, calm, and well-being, are all centred in this area. When we feel sick or frightened, when we are badly disappointed, our hearts drop. Where do they go? Into the belly. So this is a very sensitive area. If we are hurt by unkind words, we might say, 'It was like being punched in the stomach.' We have the expression, 'not having the stomach for it,' and when things go wrong we might say they have gone 'belly up'. These and many more expressions indicate the centrality of this area of our bodies in our psychic and well as physical lives.

In meditation, this area seems to be where a sense of confidence radiates from. I often use this area to focus on, experiencing it as the centre of my awareness. I have heard meditation teachers talk about completely letting go in the belly, but I am not sure that is quite right. Clearly one should relax, but there should be some strength there as well. Shunryu Suzuki comments, 'Also to gain strength in your posture, press your diaphragm towards your *hara,* or lower abdomen. This will help you maintain your physical and mental balance.' This seems to be right. It doesn't mean that when you tighten the belly it is just a sense of strength down there. As with all these things, you can experiment and see what works for you. The main thing is to become more aware of this area.

If you find it hard to relax and let go of the body while in meditation posture, you might like to lay flat on your back on the floor, with your head supported in line with the spine. You might find it easier to get a feeling for what it's like to let go in this position than in your meditation posture.

the buttocks
This is the last area I am going to mention before going on to discuss aliveness. Then we will do a meditation trying to put these three aspects of posture together. I don't have much to say about the buttocks, you might be pleased to hear, but this is another area where tensions are held and where there can be a lack of awareness. I will not quote the various expressions that relate to this area, but I am sure you can think of some that suggest being a little 'up tight'. We'll leave it at that, other than to say it is worth checking that you are not holding on to tensions there.

relaxation
The word 'relax' comes to us from the Latin *laxare*, to loosen. In other contexts it also connotes becoming less rigid, as in relaxing the rules, and letting go any effort or tension. It is also often associated with lazing around, perhaps in front of the TV with our dinner on our laps. When we relax in that sort of way we often

get up to find we are quite stiff, and we might have unconsciously been of holding a good deal of tension in our bodies. Clearly, the sort of relaxation we are looking for in our posture is rather different, and it is only possible to the extent that we have been able to align the body so that it is balanced at the pelvis and head. These two aspects are very much related to each other. If you did manage to relax completely in a non-aligned position, you would fall over. If this does not happen, you are not relaxed. Your body is holding on to something, and because this tends to be habitual it can be hard to recognize.

aliveness
This is sometimes referred to as resilience, and is compared to the ability of a tree, or a tall building, to move in the wind. If a structure is too rigid it becomes weak. It is not uncommon for people to think that their posture is rather good when in fact it is too rigid. The body is held still against itself, as it were. This might come with an exaggerated openness of the chest, as if the posture is a little puffed up. It is the sort of posture you might imagine a regimental sergeant major would adopt if he took up meditation. It might look good, but it is held together by an act of will.

The body is never still, it is a breathing living 'you'. When we talk about becoming still in meditation we do not mean it literally, only in comparison to how we are most of the time. We let the body quieten and settle, but the more this is allowed to happen, the more aware we become of the subtle feelings and movements going on in the body all the time. Most noticeably, we are breathing. It the body is aligned and relaxed we will find it easy to become aware how the body is constantly responding to our breath. The centre of gravity of the body moves as the chest expands; if we are really relaxed and attentive we might be able to feel this happening and feel the very small adjustments of the body as this happens. We might also become aware of the breath in the back, right up into the armpits. Indeed, you might sometimes have a sense of the whole body, from the feet to the crown of the head, responding to the breath. It is more of a *feeling* of movement than an actual physical movement, but it is there.

The purpose of this idea of aliveness is to encourage us to tune in to the body on a more subtle level than usual. Sitting quietly in an open and relaxed posture is an ideal opportunity to do this. To have a sense of the internal energy of the body is very helpful. To do this, begin to notice whatever is there already. Don't try to force awareness to happen, just become sensitive to your experience as it is, from one moment to the next, breath by breath. Listen to your body, adopting a receptive attitude rather than imposing ideas about what it should feel like. Just notice what is there.

meditation: listening to the body: alignment, relaxation, and aliveness

Read through this practice a few times. You don't have to follow it to the letter. Just use the overall idea as a basis for your meditation.

Spend as much time as you need to set up the posture you feel works best. If possible, get someone else to look at you and make sure you look balanced and upright, gently adjusting your head if necessary, or look in a mirror, which will at least let you see how you hold your head.

Once you have got your posture as stable as possible, let your eyes close and bring attention to your face. Notice what your face feels like and have the idea of letting your face soften. You can link this to your breathing, so there is a feeling of the face breathing and a sense of letting go on the out-breath. Imagine breathing in and out through all the pores of your face; imagine the brow becoming smooth and soft, the small muscles around your eyes relaxing. Check that you are not holding your jaw.

Spend some time becoming aware of your face, letting it soften and relax, using your breath to help maintain attention on your face, breathing in, aware of your face, breathing out, letting go of your face. Encourage a sense of the bone structure of your face, its shape, including the inside of your mouth and your tongue, which can rest gently against your upper palette just behind your front teeth. When your feel ready, let the awareness spread upwards, taking in the shape of the skull and imagining the scalp loosening against the round shape of your skull. Become aware of the crown of your head and notice any sensations there. You might imagine breathing through the crown.

Remaining aware of the crown, bring to mind the sky, as you breathe in and out. Have a sense of the limitless open space of the sky above. Imagine an attraction between the crown of your head and the sky, as if you are drawing the spacious qualities of the sky into your mind through the crown of your head on the in-breath. Then imagine that the sky exerting a subtle pull on the crown of your head, drawing it upwards on the out-breath.

Keeping this sense of being drawn upwards as attraction to the sky above you, let your awareness move down the back of your head, down your neck and down your back, until you come to the base of your spine. Now imagine the earth beneath you, feel how it supports you, sense its stability and strength, and breathe into the base of your spine.

So you are now sitting with your awareness focused on two points: the base of your spine and the crown of your head. Imagine breathing in through both of these. Imagine drawing sky energy and earth energy into your body. Then on the out-breath imagine the earth drawing the base of your spine down towards the centre of the earth, while at the same time the sky draws the crown of your head upward into limitless spaciousness.

Just sit there being aware of the breath, aware of the earth and the sky, aware of a subtle attraction between these two points of your body and these two fundamental elements. Imagine drawing the qualities of these elements into your body: the spaciousness of the sky, the stability of the earth. Imagine your body coming into alignment, your head finding its natural balance on your spine, your pelvis making any slight adjustments, the neck lengthening and softening, the shoulders releasing.

Breathe your back, its breadth and its length. Have a sense of the back of your body breathing and very gently expanding in all directions, a sense that there is all the room in the world for you. Breathe your back, remaining aware of the sky and the earth. Breathe the muscles and the spine. Imagine the spine alive inside your body, made up of soft tissue, nerves, and bones; imagine it full of impulses, electric in your body. Imagine that through your spine the sky and the earth come into relationship, the sky father, the earth mother. Breathing your back, let it soften, lengthen, broaden. Enjoy sitting in communion with these two great elements. Let them support and enliven you, draw into your body the energy of the earth and the cosmos.

When you feel the time is right, let your awareness spread through the pelvis, into the bones of your pelvis, including your sexual organs. Now breathe down into the legs, letting go, releasing the muscles, giving the weight of those big bones to the earth for support. Breathe the delicate bones of the feet, let the soles of your feet soften.

When you feel ready, move up the front of the body, taking in the belly, and feel how it breathes. Be aware how the ribcage moves, feel how it opens to receive the breath. Let the breath very gently lift and open the chest around your heart. Take your time, don't push. Have a sense of the awareness, like a soft golden light spreading throughout your body. Then, moving up the body, move the awareness into the arms, through the muscles and bones and down into the hands. Let the awareness gather in the hands for a while, let it soften and enliven the hands, let a sense of kindness fill your hands. Then slowly let your awareness move back into your whole body, sitting with a sense of your whole body breathing, alive with the breath. Remember the earth and the sky, then just relax. Sit for a while without trying to do anything; nothing at all. Just sit with things as they are, making no effort to control your experience.

3

the world and the body

> *The way through the world is more difficult to find
> than the way beyond it.*
> Wallace Stevens[5]

According to the story that has been handed down to us,[6] the Buddha gained 'enlightenment' beneath a large spreading bodhi tree. This tree has beautiful leaves, like giant inverted teardrops. The story of the period leading up to the Buddha's enlightenment is very rich in symbolism, much of which evokes the earth and the feminine. The Buddha-to-be, Prince Siddhartha, seems to have been a very determined young man, so determined that he brought himself to the verge of death by practising serve austerities with a small group of fellow ascetics.

It seems that this band of brothers was convinced that the liberation they sought could be achieved by overcoming all attachments and concern for their physical welfare. This sort of thinking is quite common in religious traditions, which see the spiritual as somehow in opposition to the worldly. The spirit is trapped inside the body, or sometimes the mind is opposed to the body. This is a form of dualism that runs like a seam of lead through religious and philosophical traditions of both East and West. In ancient India it was a very common belief. This was a time of great 'spiritual' seeking, so it was not uncommon to find groups of men – it was nearly always men – doing the most awful things to themselves in order to liberate the spirit from what they considered the prison of their bodies. Some of these involved deprivation of the most extreme sought. I've put 'spiritual' in quotation marks as it is a word I don't like very much, but I will say more about that later.

We are told that the emaciated prince went into a river to bathe, but having got in he was so weak that he couldn't get out, and he thought he might be swept away. This episode caused him to reconsider his attempts at liberation. He somehow managed to haul himself out of the river, be he realized that if he continued his self-torture he would soon be dead. He found himself in a rather difficult position, for we are told that he had become quite famous for his ascetic practices. Holy men who did this sort of thing were much revered. As well as being a local celebrity he was the acknowledged leader of the little band with whom he lived in the forest. They looked up to him and expected him to find liberation very soon. This all sounds a bit extreme, but spiritual quests are apt to go that way. Unfortunately, it seems that fanaticism even to the point of death is not uncommon. We still hear of 'religious groups' committing suicide, in the belief that through such action, salvation of one sort or another may be found.

So there he was, this still quite young man, who had renounced a kingdom in order to find the answer to life's suffering, faced with the prospect of giving up. Sometimes it takes great strength of character to realize that we have taken the wrong path, particularly in the face of losing status and the approval of those we are close to. It seems, however, that Siddhartha was determined to find liberation and, having become convinced of the folly of his previous attempts, he was willing to suffer the taunts of others. He had realized that if he were to die, his search would end and all his effort would have been completely wasted. He had already left his family, including an infant son, and disappointed his father by renouncing the throne. In addition he had practised with renowned spiritual masters of the age.

Siddhartha had nearly met his end in the river, and he realized that his self-mortification had brought him nothing except the prospect of a early death. He decided he would have to attend to his bodily needs if he wanted to continue seeking the end of suffering. He took leave of his fellow ascetics, who refused to listen to his pleas that they too should give up their self-imposed sufferings.

What happened next seems to have both a prosaic and symbolic meaning. He met a young woman who offered him some food. There are differing accounts of this time before the prince's enlightenment, but I rather like this particular version. It does not seem too fanciful to me to see this as the feminine aspect coming back into the picture, an aspect that had been excluded from his ascetic period. It is a moving picture: this emaciated young man, dressed in a few rags, rejected by his friends, emerging from the forest and encountering this young woman who offers him nourishment. We can see this as suggesting the importance of attending to our everyday needs – taking care of ourselves. To me it is also a warning that we should not place the 'spiritual life' in opposition to the worldly life.

This, then, is the start of a kind of healing for the young prince; a healing of his abused body, and also a psychical healing, in which the necessity of the nurturing aspects of the psyche is acknowledged. I want to labour this point a little as I find that many people who take up meditation and other 'spiritual' practices do so in a rather hard way, as though they are not good enough and they need to overcome themselves in order to improve. It is easy to become wilful in trying to make ourselves 'better'. The story I have told is a very extreme example of this sort of willed effort, but I know a lot of people who, in trying to improve themselves, realize they have become cut off from what we might call their feminine aspect. In their praiseworthy attempts to make progress, they have left something of themselves behind, they have forgotten simply to care for themselves, forgotten to nourish themselves so that they can practise openly and lovingly. When we take up a spiritual path, we need to take care that we do not repress aspects of ourselves such as our sexuality and our maternal or paternal urges. We are in danger of doing this if we become too idealistic and ignore the emotional side of our experience.

Our story is getting a little long with these detours, but these sorts of stories, that have filtered down the ages, are so full of interesting incidents that they provoke reflection, and it seems worth highlighting various aspects.

To continue with the story, Siddhartha accepts from the young woman some rice cooked in milk. Of course in reality it must have taken him a while to get his body back into shape, as we are told that he had grown so thin that he could feel his backbone through his belly. So perhaps the young woman brought him food every day for some weeks and took care of him. There is a related incident that I want to mention here. This is sometimes said to have happened before he left his fellow ascetics, so it is part of the realization that he had gone rather badly astray, though in other accounts it takes place a little later. Whenever it happened, it is significant. It is sometimes called the rose-apple experience. Trees seem to play a big part in this myth and I will say a little more about that later.

We are told that Siddhartha remembered sitting under a rose-apple tree as a young boy, watching his father plough a field. Some people have questioned why a king should be ploughing, and some claim that it was a ritual ploughing, but it does seem that our idea of a king is rather different from the ruler of a small province in ancient India. Siddhartha is sitting under this tree and suddenly he finds himself suffused with pleasure and tranquillity. He is what we might now call 'blissed out'. Recalling this incident seems to have got the him thinking that perhaps the way forward had something to do with accepting the pleasure that can arise when one is relaxed and free from anxiety and craving. This story contains another image of the feminine, for the earth is being turned, and all that implies in the sense of cultivation and dependence on the earth.

It is significant that Siddhartha sits under a tree in this incident, for this prefigures his enlightenment, when we again find him sitting under a tree, this time the vast spreading bodhi tree at a place which is now called Bodh Gaya, where a bodhi tree, said to be a third generation of the very tree under which the Buddha sat, grows today and is a place of pilgrimage.

So we find ourselves back at the bodhi tree. I want to say a little about trees before describing another incident about the Buddha's enlightenment. Trees crop up in many of the world's great stories, for example in one of the earliest stories, that of Gilgamesh. No one knows just how old this story is, but we do know that it was first written down around 2100 BCE in cuneiform text on clay tablets in what is now Iraq. So it makes even the story of the Buddha seem relatively recent. One of the principal incidents involves Gilgamesh, a semi-divine king of Urak, who is travelling with his companion Enkidu to cut down a sacred cedar of Lebanon to make the temple gate for Urak. The forest is protected by a magical figure, Humbaba, who is killed by Enkidu and the tree taken. This act of

51

hubris foreshadows the death of Enkidu, a death that plunges Gilgamesh into despair. So trees were sometimes regarded as sacred this far into the past.

The world tree, Yggdrasil, is central in Norse mythology as symbolic of both time and of life, while the tree in Christian mythology is found both in the Garden of Eden, as the tree of knowledge, and as the cross, thus becoming a central motif. There are many other examples of the importance of the tree as a symbol. Trees have clearly been of great use to humankind, as a provider of food, construction materials, and all sorts of vehicles and implements, but I don't think the utilitarian nature of the tree explains its prominence in stories and myths. It is rather that humankind is moved by trees.

Standing near a mature oak, for instance, one has an immediate sense of why this tree was so important to the pagans of England. Something about such trees calls to us. It's partly to do with their great age in relation to ourselves. Trees often strike me as a slow kind of magic; it is a wonder that such magnificent living things can grow from a tiny seed in an alchemy of sun, rain, and earth. Trees are also revered because they seem to unite the elements of earth and sky, which represent the two basic forces experienced by humankind. Whether they are known by the names of the old gods, or more abstractly as yin and yang, the masculine and the feminine, these are the two basic archetypal images of human culture. The earth represents the body, just as the sky can represent the mind; the earth, our feeling and sensations, the sky, our intellect and vision. The branches of the tree reach towards the sky, while its roots, which are often imagined as extensive as its branches, go down into the earth. The tree brings together, unites, the sky and earth, the father-mother. Moreover, the tree draws on the nourishment of both the sun and the earth. It is no coincidence that the Buddha gained his profound insight into the nature of reality seated on the earth under the shade of the great spreading branches of the bodhi tree.

There is one more episode from the Buddha's quest that I want to mention. I find it the most moving of all the events in the mythology of the Buddha's life, perhaps because it is so central to the spirit of how I understand the practice of meditation, indeed, the whole of the Buddhist approach to life.

Before I recount this, perhaps I should say a little about what I mean when I use this term 'mythology'. It is sometimes used rather dismissively, which is quite contrary to the meaning that I associate with it. I understand it to refer to events and stories with meaning. Myths are stories or ways of understanding events that have a deep resonance in the human mind. While I was writing about the symbolism of trees and mentioned Norse mythology, I could not help but pause, for my mind became flooded with the story of Sigurd (Siegfried), which I encountered in a picture book as a young child. Myths have a kind of condensed form that means they remain with us, they are full of a symbolism that is never exhausted, and we find ourselves returning to them again and again for a sense of meaning. Although we might be only dimly aware of them, we all have our own myths which inform the way we go through the world, and the way we understand our past and give us hope, or dread, for our future. I hope that gives you a sense of how I am using the word. The other thing about mythology is that it can never really be pinned down or fully explained. The meaning of myths changes with the experience that we bring to them.

The incident I want to say a little about is known as the calling of the earth to witness. That is rather a splendid phrase. In western culture we are more likely to say, 'Let God be my witness,' but the Buddha called on the earth because, on the very brink of enlightenment, he was challenged by a figure known in Buddhism as Mara. Now Mara, which is a rather pretty name for this ugly character, is a kind of Buddhist devil. He is usually more of an irritation to the Buddha than a threat, but in this case he does make a good stab at preventing the Buddha attaining enlightenment. I want to quote here from the *Lalitavistara*, a poetic version of the life of the Buddha as recorded in the Mahayana tradition.

calling the earth to witness

> The Bodhisattva touched himself on the forehead with his right hand, and Mara fled toward the south, thinking: 'The Bodhisattva has a sword in his hand!' But then he thought: 'There was nothing!' and again turned back.
>
> Mara aimed at the Bodhisattva all sorts of frightening weapons: swords, arrows, lances, javelins, stones, spindles, axes, rammers, sharp lightning bolts, clubs, discuses, hammers, uprooted trees,

*boulders, chains and iron balls. But no sooner did he
throw these weapons than they changed into
garlands and canopies of flowers. Flowers covered
the ground and hung as ornaments for the tree of
wisdom. So magnificent were these displays made
for the Bodhisattva that Mara ... was devoured with
anger and envy. He cried to the Bodhisattva: 'Arise!
Arise, youthful prince! Go and enjoy your
kingdom! Through what merit will you gain
deliverance?'*

Then he addressed the Bodhisattva with this verse.

*In a previous existence,
I freely made an irreproachable offering;
to this you are the witness;
but you have no witness to offer evidence in your
    support,
and so you will be conquered!*

*The Bodhisattva replied: '... this earth is my wit-
ness.' And the Bodhisattva enveloped Mara and all
his following with a thought proceeding from love
and compassion. He was like a lion, without distress
or fear, terror or weakness, without dejection, without confusion, without agitation, without the dread
which makes the hair stand on end.
With his right hand ... he touched all parts of his
body and then gently touched the earth. And at that
moment he uttered this verse:*

*This earth, the home of all beings,
is impartial and free of malice
toward everything which moves or does not move.*

Here is the guarantee that there is no deception:
Take the earth as my witness.

And as the Bodhisattva touched the great earth, it
trembled in six ways: it trembled, trembled
strongly, trembled strongly on all sides. Re-
sounded, resounded strongly, resounded strongly
on all sides. Just as the bronze bells from Magadha
ring out when struck with a stick, so this great earth
resounded and resounded again when touched by
the hand of the Bodhisattva.

Then the goddess of the earth,... the goddess named
Sthavara, surrounded by a following of a hundred
times ten million earth goddesses, shook the whole
great earth. Not far from the Bodhisattva, she re-
vealed the upper half of her body adorned with all its
ornaments, and bowing with joined palms, spoke
thus to the Bodhisattva: 'Just so, Great Beings. It is
indeed as you have declared! We appear here to at-
test to it. Moreover, O Bhagavat, you yourself have
become the supreme witness of both the human and
god realms. In truth, you are the purest of all
beings.'...

Having heard the voice from the earth,
the deceiver and his army, terrified and broken,
began to flee. Like foxes in the woods
who hear the lion's roar,
like crows at the full of a clump of earth,
all suddenly dispersed.[7]

What I like best about this story is not the makeshift
weapons, but being told that the Bodhisattva – which
means a being of great compassion – touches all parts

of his body before gently touching the earth. It is this powerful invocation of the earth that most strikes me, for it seems that Buddhism and meditation, through which the Buddha gained his insight, is brought down to earth.

I began this chapter with a short quote from a poem by Wallace Stevens, 'The way through the world is more difficult to find than the way beyond it,' and it seems to me that this calling of the earth to witness confirms that Buddhism and meditation are concerned with 'the way through the world'. That is to say, it is a wholly human affair, which includes our bodies and our hearts, as well as our minds. Touching the earth, calling the earth to witness, evokes, in the strongest possible way, the feminine principle, in the form of the earth goddess. In symbolic terms, the feminine is associated with the body, with the unconscious, with what happens below the level of the ego and the rational mind. It relates to the emotions, the heart, and the soul in contrast to the spirit.

The myth of the Buddha's enlightenment marks the start of the tradition of Buddhist meditation as the direct path to insight. It seems to me that mythology and the body are related in a number of important respects. Both are somewhat indistinct, they don't remain the same. They both have to do with what lies below the surface, under the skin. And the body and mythology have two characteristics that seem at first to be contradictory. They speak to us directly and they speak to us through the imagination. While we might think of the imagination as something involved in day-dreaming or vague and unformed thoughts, this is not what I mean. Imagination is our innate ability to form images; not necessarily visual images, but any sort of representation. In particular, and at it most basic, imagination allows us a sense of ourselves: to have an emotional, feeling sense of who and how we are. Thus it is through the imagination, in this sense, that we have awareness of the body, and indeed of other people and the world. While our senses supply us with raw data, it is the imagination that gives this data meaning and form.

I want now to describe a meditation practice that uses our imagination and some of the other things I have spoken about. As with all the meditations in this book, I suggest you read through it a couple of times, then sit in a good posture and just see what happens. Don't feel you should follow what I say in a machine-like fashion, just use it to spark your imagination and take an interest in your response.

meditation: letting the earth support us

> *Sitting in meditation posture, take as much time as you need to get comfortable and allow the body to settle. Begin by just becoming aware of the sounds around you. Don't strain to hear; just notice any noises. Have a sense of the world around you, a sense of human life and the natural world. If you are in a town, let your imagination expand beyond the suburbs into the surrounding countryside. Imagine all that activity around you, so that you are aware that you are sitting in the midst of life. Have a sense of how all that life arises from, and is supported by, the world.*

Keeping this sense of the world, come to your breath. Be aware that in this simple act of breathing you are sustaining and nourishing your life. Be aware that every time you breathe you are taking in the world around you. What was outside you is drawn into your body as you breathe. The miracle of your body takes what it needs and gives back to the outside world what it doesn't use. Aware of your own breath, be aware of the breathing world all around you. The human beings, animals, and plants all breathing in their individual way, all sustained by the biosphere just as you are being sustained.

See if you can imagine the whole of your body breathing, every cell. Breathe into the bones and the organs, imagining the whole surface of your skin breathing in and out as you breathe in and out of your lungs. Think of the whole world breathing.

Keeping this sense of a breathing body in a breathing world, be aware of your contact with the ground. Become aware how it feels to be in contact with the earth through your body. Try to have a sense of giving the weight of your body to the ground, at the same time maintaining a sound posture. The more you can give the body to the ground for support, the easier it will be to sit well, as long as your posture is balanced. If you are sitting indoors, allow yourself to be aware that under the building is the earth. You might like to remember that the earth was there before the building, and may at some time be uncovered again. Think of the earth spreading out beneath you, think of all the life that the earth has supported throughout time. See if you can have a sense of the earth supporting you as it supports all life, taking your weight, accepting you as you are, holding your body unconditionally. With each out-breath, give your weight more and more to the earth, have a feeling of the supporting earth, the covering sky, and the living world all around you. Just be present, with a sense of having taken your place in the world and that the world is on your side.

4

the breathing body

Before we are born, we develop inside our mothers. Our world is located inside another being; we are totally dependent on them. Once we are born, although we are still more or less totally dependent on our carers, we enter a different relationship with the world around us. We enter the world, we start to breathe, and from that first moment the world also enters us. We suck the world into our bodies in our instinctive desire to be part of this world. This relationship of direct dependence on the world continues until we die. This is so everyday that we rarely notice it or reflect on it. We often find the world quite a difficult place. Sometimes we feel we don't belong. We might experience isolation or loneliness, or feel out of place. When we have these feelings, we are forgetting our fundamental connection with the world. We separate ourselves from the world because we are unhappy, but the world is still there, not only all around us, but also inside us. The world continues to sustain us, moment-to-moment, through our breathing.

the body

Among other things, meditation offers us a chance to experience our connection with the world, to allow a sense of intimate belonging to arise in our bodies. Although I say 'arise', it is ever-present as far as the body is concerned. It is more that meditation presents an opportunity to notice and to remember. While our connection to the world, through which we gain our sense of well-being and meaning, is normally very complex, it is very psychological in the sense that it is dominated by our ego. Because it is complex and dependent on keeping our ego happy, it is always fragile. A harsh word, a little disappointment, and we start to feel the world has let us down, and our sense of self-worth is threatened. In meditation it is possible to have a different sense of what it means to be in the world, a sense that is not based on the unsatisfiable demands of the ego – the constant thinking, judging, and calculation – but a feeling sense that arises naturally when we pay kind attention to our breath and our bodies.

If you have spent any time with a dead body, you might have been struck by just how lifeless it is. I know that sounds like a strange thing to say, but that is how I experience them. In many ways, they are the same as they were before they died. Although the person has gone, the body is still there and it looks much the same as it did the moment before it took its last breath. It is easy to see why most religions claim that the body and the soul – and here I am using 'soul' in its more conventional sense – are different things, different stuff. When you are with the dead, they are just too dead. It is as though whatever made the person alive has gone somewhere else, because for something simply to vanish is outside our usual experience. Things do not just disappear, so they must have gone somewhere. The life that is no longer there must, we think – or rather we feel – have gone somewhere else.

I don't intend to go into the various beliefs, Buddhist or otherwise, on what might happen after we die. I just want to make the simple point that although we tend to think of life as a property of an individual, that was never really the case, or at least that isn't the whole story. If we understand life to be a property of a particular person, we become confused over where that life has gone after that person dies. One moment it is there, and the next it has completely disappeared. But life is never something that is somehow only inside of us. Our bodies are not as discrete as that. We have never for a moment existed as something other than the world. I tend to feel (for it is more a matter of feeling than thought) that what we experience as a individual is also just the world expressing itself in a particular form. Do you have a sense of what I mean? It is as though there is a field of life, of energy, constantly throwing up unique expressions of itself, like ocean waves. But the waves are still ocean; they rise and fall and the ocean is still there. We come and go, but life, the ocean that we are, is still there. We begin to have a sense of ourselves as world, but when someone dies it doesn't seem quite so cut and dried. The world of which they were a part is still there, and therefore there is a sense in which they are still there, at least, the part of them that was the world is still

the body

there. It is not easy to explain what I mean, because it is not really an idea but a particular sense of being in the world, in which we also intuit that the world is within us as much as we are within the world. When I scattered my father's ashes in a place that he loved, I felt I was returning him to the earth, and this was somehow an acknowledgement of life in death.

It is through our breath that we can most directly cultivate a sense of being in the world. The breath does not really need us, in terms of how we normally experience ourselves. The breath is far too vital an activity to entrust to the ego. It seems to me there has been a strange reversal in the way we think of ourselves. Perhaps we can partly blame Descartes, whose famous dictum, 'I think therefore I am,' has tricked us into thinking ourselves into existence. Descartes wanted to see what remained if there was a demon tricking him into thinking that he had a body, and that this body existed in a world. He concluded that the only thing that he could not doubt, given the presumed activity of his demonic friend, was that he thought. That is to say, his thought was a self-validating experience.

As a piece of philosophical reasoning, Descartes deserves credit. What makes this interesting is that the demon was his own mind. While the notion that thought proves one's existence appeals to the thinking ego, from the point of view of the body the ego is irrelevant. The body is not dependent on the ego for its existence, but the ego is entirely dependent on the body. When, during meditation, you move the weight of your awareness from all those thoughts to the experience of possessing a living, breathing body, there is a sense of relief, and we start to realize that we get on quite well without all that frantic mental activity. It really is OK to relax into your sense of your body, your heart beating, your organs getting on with their work, your blood taking oxygen around your body, your lungs inhaling and expelling the air. There is a whole universe of life within, and it all gets on quite nicely without 'you'.

There is a story that does the rounds in the Buddhist world about a meeting between two Buddhist big-wigs, a Zen master and a Tibetan guru, that took place at Harvard about thirty years ago.[8] The Zen master began by flourishing an orange and asking the Tibetan, 'What is this? What is this?' He was clearly ready to pounce on whatever answer was presented. The whole thing was taking place through translators, but the Tibetan appeared not to understand. The Zen master demanded even more forcibly, 'What is this?' Looking a little puzzled, the Tibetan asked his translator, 'Don't they have oranges where he comes from?'

The mind, in terms of the ego, has a tendency to make things very complex. It is, as Descartes demonstrated, quite capable of thinking itself to the edge of self-negation, though it always turns back at the last moment, because its overriding concern is its own existence. The Zen master was trying to make a valid point in inviting the Tibetan to question the assumed existence of things outside of ourselves. But the Tibetan was happy for the orange to be an orange. It is not that he was right, it is just another way of looking. What I am suggesting is that in meditation we can relax the mind a little and relate to our experience directly and simply. An orange can be an orange.

There is a confusion, I feel, between awareness and thought. We tend to think that awareness is dependent on thought, whereas the opposite is true. Awareness does not need thought, but thought does need awareness. Thinking is something we do with our awareness. It is an activity associated with the fact that we are aware. For instance, if you put your hand on a hot surface, your experience is that you think it is hot and you quickly withdraw your hand. But if that were the case you would be burned, because thinking takes a relatively long time. What happens is that the body feels the heat and instantly reacts. It is hard-wired into us, to use a modern expression; it has nothing to do with thought. What then happens is quite fascinating. The brain has the ability to make you believe that the thought that the surface was hot preceded your taking your hand away, when in fact you took your hand away well before you had any conscious awareness of the experience of heat. This is a very strange thing. It is a kind of time warp in the mind, in which the conscious experience of knowing something is put back in time to give the impression that you felt the heat and withdrew your hand because you 'knew' it was hot. This happens not only with hot surfaces, but all the time. One is tricked into experiencing consciousness as being causal although it actually follows an action. This is something to think about. Your ability to perform many complex activities, such as a sport or a skill, is not dependent on thought in a conscious sense. The body learns to do these things without the aid of the thinking mind.

Meditation gives us the opportunity to think a little less. Although this can be difficult at first, in time we learn to trust our experience in a different way. We find we don't have to make everything so complicated, that a feeling can be just a feeling, a thought can be just a thought; it doesn't have to be elaborated upon, it doesn't have to become the concern of the ego. The breath and the body are the best places to begin to develop this direct experience of ourselves. The body is aware in ways we are not conscious of. When we start to become more consciously aware of our breath and our body we find a whole world of sensation, feeling, emotion, and, indeed, thought of which we were previously unaware. It is as though there is a whole universe of the experiencing body that we do not normally notice.

Take a moment now to become aware of your hands. Notice whether they are warm or cold. Notice that in this moment they are full of sensations. Notice how you can feel your life energy in them. These feelings are always there in your hands, but the conscious mind, which can process only a small amount of information at a time, is too busy to notice. Of course, it is interesting that we can think about things, but if we spend all our time doing it, we start to lose touch with ourselves, become lost in the world of our own thoughts, and increasingly fail to notice the world inside and outside our ego-centred minds. We become trapped in a self-created world of our own egos.

Just breathing with awareness brings us into a direct feeling relationship with the world inside and outside our own bodies. But our minds are so accustomed to thinking, that the simple direct awareness of the body doesn't satisfy it. We find we are off somewhere else, often into our fantasies or anxieties. When this happens we need to remind ourselves that the breath and the body are still there. Unlike our minds, they have not gone anywhere. So although we are constantly distracted, we try to develop a sense of confidence in the presence of the breathing body. There are times when we become aware of our distractions and realize that we have been lost in our thoughts. If we have a basic confidence in the presence of our bodies, we will find we can bring our awareness back to this direct experience of ourselves during those moments of awareness.

The body and the breath provide the foundations for meditation. Without these foundations there will be no stability in our practice. Without this awareness we are homeless. Without somewhere to return to, we wander aimlessly. But once we have cultivated a feeling sense of our bodies, we always have a home to come back to. Even though our minds still wander, they will find their way home.

meditation: the breathing body

> *Take up your meditation posture, carefully taking your time to get comfortable, bearing in mind that this is also part of the practice. Once you have settled, come to your breath. At first, just become aware when you are breathing in and when you are breathing out. Apply*

only the effort you need to be aware of your breathing, saying to yourself, 'breathing in, breathing out,' as you do so. I suggest that from the start you make a commitment to being aware of your breath and exert the effort needed, even if it feels a little crude to begin with. Once you have tuned in to the breath, use it to scan the whole of your body, so if you start at your face, say to yourself, 'Breathing in, I am aware of my face; breathing out, I am aware of my face.' Move down your whole body in this way. You can do this in any order that feels natural, but do not move on until you feel you have made some contact with the part of the body you are focusing on. Where there is greater sensitivity, such as your face and hands, go into a little more detail. If you notice tension in parts of your body, you might try saying, 'Breathing in, I am aware of my shoulders; breathing out, I soften my shoulders,' or any other phrase that feels right to you, as long as it includes the conscious acknowledgement that you are breathing with each breath.

Once you have proceeded through your whole body in this way, focus on the parts that are directly affected by your breath. This will include the belly and the chest, and also the back. Do this by saying to yourself something like, 'Breathing in, I feel my chest open; breathing out, I feel my chest fall,' again choosing words you feel comfortable with. Find an encouraging and kindly internal voice. You can let this internal voice soften and quieten once you feel more engaged. It needs to be just strong enough to hold your attention; it is giving your thinking mind something to do.

Next, move from stating what is happening on a physical level to allowing yourself to experience what is happening on a feeling level. So you might say something like, 'Breathing in, my belly feels …; breathing out, my belly feels….' Keep saying this with whatever words come to you; rather than 'think' of the words, just let them arise. We are not trying to impose an idea of how our body feels, but to let the words arise from the body. Do not censor what comes up, even if it is a little strange. 'Breathing in, my heart feels like red, a balloon, a house, a wet cat, a loaf of bread, heavy, a spy….' If it changes, let it change. Although I suggest using words, it might be an image that arises, and that is fine. Adapt what you are saying to fit what is happening. Do this with whatever parts of your body you wish, parts that feel they have something to say, as it were. I usually make sure I include the genitals, belly, heart area, face, and hands, plus any other areas that feel they could benefit from the attention of a kind breath.

When you feel ready, return to a general awareness of the whole body, saying to yourself something like, 'Breathing in, I am aware of my body; breathing out, I am aware of my body.' Then gently imagine your awareness remaining within your body but also beginning to take in what is around you. Start with what you are sensually aware of. 'Breathing in, I feel the air touching my face; breathing out, I feel the ground under my feet.' Then extend your imagination: 'Breathing in, I am aware of the room around me. Breathing out, I am aware of the room around me. Breathing in, I am aware of the street outside,' and so on. Imagine your awareness spreading into the world, and see what comes to mind. Include people, trees, animals, linking them all to your breath. Then, when you have a sense of the world around you, say to yourself something like, 'Breathing in the world, breathing out the world.' Breathe out, and let the words gradually fade away, so you are sitting with a sense of your breathing body in a breathing world. To bring the meditation to a close, relax your effort completely and sit for a while, no longer trying to do anything at all, just sitting with your experience as it is in the moment.

the mindfulness of breathing

The mindfulness of breathing is one of the first of the meditation practices we find in the *Satipatthana Sutta*. This sutta offers a progressive extension of mindfulness, starting with the breath and the body, through feeling and emotions, to thoughts, and then what are called the *dharmas*. I will talk about this final type of meditation later, when I address the relationship between the body and insight. The fact that the sutta, which is a meditators' manual, starts with cultivation of awareness of the breath, indicates its importance. It seems such a simple thing to sit still and notice that you are breathing. But although it is very simple, it can prove quite difficult.

There are different versions of this practice, but they usually start with counting one's breaths. We sit there, breathing normally, and begin to count our breaths. To start with, we count at the end of the out-breath: breathing in, breathing out, count one; breathing in, breathing out, count two. We continue in this way until we have counted ten breaths, and then we start again from one.

When people learn this meditation, they often take the point of the practice to be counting the breaths, but this is not the case. The counting in this stage and the next should be understood merely as an aid to staying with our breaths. This sounds very simple, but it is all too easy for counting the breaths to become the focus of the meditation rather than the breath itself. The counting offers something of a bridge from a conceptual to what we might call a more meditative mode of awareness. Counting gives the more conceptual part of our mind something to do, which is connected with the breath. It is a little hook that we put at the end or the beginning of our breaths to help the mind remain with our experience of breathing. However, if we make the counting the point of the practice, the experience of being with our breath becomes rather dry and mechanical, and we can lose the sense of aliveness that this simple abiding with our breath offers us.

The question arises as to whether counting the breaths is therefore a useful aid to the practice. In the *Satipatthana Sutta* we are not told to count the breaths, only to be aware what type of breath each is: long or short, shallow or deep. This is also the case in the *Anapassati Sutta*, another important early text on meditation. In both these suttas, we are encouraged to be aware of the quality of the breath, noticing whether it is fine or course, for instance. Counting seems to have entered the practice in various commentaries on these original sources. The point seems to be to judge, through honest attention to your own experience of counting, whether you find that helpful in promoting a sense of intimacy with the breath.

From personal experience of this practice over some twenty years, I have found counting the breaths to be very helpful, but I have met a number of people for whom it seems to cause a certain amount of anxiety. It seems to make the practice into something that they can fail at, and rather than enjoying being with their breath, they find the whole process something of an ordeal. If you also find this, try focusing on the quality of the breath in the body.

This leads us into a more general area of to what extent one should feel free to deviate from the standard form of any meditation practice. The answer touches on a distinction between what we might call the spirit and the letter. The meditator needs a sense of what it feels like to be increasingly aware of the body through mindfulness of the breath. This feeling for the practice is developed over years of practice. It is not a static feeling, but deepens and changes in relation to our experience. In order to trust your intuition, there has to be a body of experience that forms the background that your intuition draws upon. On the other hand, there has to be a certain willingness to trust in what feels right in order to build up that body of experience. If we always approach our meditation in the same way, it will take us a long time to learn what works for us.

So there is no simple answer that you should always do this or that. In the end, meditation is a very individual experience and no one can really tell you what you should do. The important thing is to try, as far as possible, to develop a clear sense of what is happening when you meditate. If you spent twenty minutes thinking about work or romance, and didn't really notice the breath at all, just admit that to yourself. It is not that it is wrong, but it is not meditation. It would, however, be meditation if, between experiencing the anxiety about work, or your sadness over a lost love, you came back to the breath in your body whenever you had little windows of awareness. It might even be that you start to make a connection between what your mind is thinking about and how your body and breath feels. It is in this connection between our predominately mental experience, or thinking, and our bodily experience, or feeling, that the breath is so important, for it is through awareness of our breathing body that the mental and the sensational are brought together. It is in this feeling of a kind of coming together that the spirit of the practice is to be found. If you are anxious about work, you should be aware of that, but perhaps you can also begin to notice what this anxiety feels like in your body, in the belly perhaps, or around the heart area. Ask yourself how you are breathing this experience. We will look further into this in the following chapter.

We have a tendency to talk about the breath as if it is a thing. I find myself doing this. I might suggest being aware of the breath, but this is rather a lazy way to talk, and it can be a bit misleading. In the first place, it is your breath, not some abstract thing. It is the most vital activity of your body. We are never really aware of the breath as an abstract thing. What we are aware of is our breathing body. This seems to me to have a different feel to it. Becoming aware of your breathing body is quite an intimate thing to try to do. It sounds rather different from being aware of the breath. There is no breath without the body and no body without the breath. The breath defines the body. Without the breath, the body as a living thing ceases to be. It is a dead body, which is a very different thing to a living one. Breathing is not just something that the body does, it is the body.

5

the body and the heart

I have suggested a connection between the body, the imagination, and what I have called soul. I will explain later why I have chosen this rather ambiguous term; for now, it is enough to know that I do not mean something other than body, or something that continues after the body dies, or indeed any sort of 'thing'. I mean a quality, as when we say someone or something has soul. Soul is the quality that connects us with others and the world. In this sense, soul is not individual but partakes of a world soul. It arises from an awareness of our limitations and our vulnerability. It might not, then, be very attractive at first sight. We like the idea of being independent, we don't like the idea that we are dependent on others, we find it hard to acknowledge how fragile we are. Many people, I believe, take up a spiritual practice because they are looking for more control over their lives. They are looking to feel more powerful and independent. Meditation appeals to them because it seems to offer a way of rising above it all, gaining mastery over oneself and those uncomfortable feelings. It is often equated with gaining control over the darker sides of ourselves, the parts we don't want the world to see. It is therefore a little ironic that, in practice, meditation does the very opposite. What we gradually realize, through the practice of meditation, is the complex and interrelated nature of our own being. What is perhaps the biggest surprise is that the more we understand and experience this sense of connection and dependence on the world, the less we feel threatened and frightened by it.

When we first learn a meditation like the loving-kindness meditation,[9] we might think it is going to help us to become a very kind and compassionate person. Behind this wish is also the idea that it will bring a end to difficult feelings, such as a lack of self-worth, and that we will learn to love ourselves and others and everything will be well in the world. But the self that we want to learn to love is often an idealized self. We might have an image of ourselves going beyond anger and self-pity, a perfectly content and loving human being, free of irritation, jealousy, and hatred. We think we will become like a Buddha; after all, isn't that what Buddhism is about?

If you have been around Buddhists for any length of time, you will know that this is quite laughable. Although when you go to a meditation class it is all too easy to project these ideas onto the teacher, don't be fooled. In all likelihood they are in the same a mess as you. What then, you might quite fairly ask, is the point of meditation? It is not unlike Socrates' claim that he knew that he knew nothing, and it was in his awareness of his own ignorance that his wisdom was to be found. When we meditate, we begin to have intimations of what lies below the surface. We start to get a different sense of ourselves that is not so dominated by our ego sense. It is not that our ego goes away; it is still calculating and scheming, looking to assert or protect itself. The difference is that we slowly begin to see that this is what it is always doing.

To return to our story, Siddhartha is on the point of gaining enlightenment when he is assailed by Mara. We could interpret this as the ego trying to resist the breakthrough he is about to make. Siddhartha, however, does not offer any resistance, he just lets Mara be. He touches the earth to bring alive his connection with the world. The response of the earth is to support him. We might start to meditate because we want to become a perfect Buddha, but after a while we begin to notice that what we are already is quite interesting, that it is possible to sit with our difficult thoughts and feelings, those feelings of not being good enough. We start to notice that, yes, they are there, coming and going, but so are the sensations in our body, so is the feeling of being supported by the earth, so is the wide sky above us. And after a while, we develop confidence that we can sit with the whole of our experience as it unfolds, and we don't have to censor it or avoid it in any way. We might even find that we begin to welcome it. When we feel irritation, we notice that it brings with it a sense of energy. Perhaps the physical sensations that accompany our irritation are not so bad. Instead of desperately trying to justify our irritation, we just breathe it, we just stay with whatever sense we have of our bodies and our breath, and we notice that it passes. The next time it comes along we feel a little different about it; we might even feel a sense of kindness towards it, and feel less of a need to deal with it in some way. We are a little easier about just sitting with it and letting it exhaust itself.

Awareness of the body offers us a sense of stability. This stability is both literal and imaginative. It is literal in the sense of the posture, and imaginative in the sense that we can cultivate a feeling of connection with the world and allow that sense of connection to support and sustain our practice. The physical and imaginative aspects of our posture are not separate, for how we hold our body has a profound effect on our mind. Become aware of how you are sitting now, and see if you can feel how your posture and your mental states are intimately related. This is true all the time, not just when we meditate. The Zen tradition, which stresses meditation and posture, is very aware of this body-mind relationship. Shunryu Suzuki has this to say about the posture.

> *These forms are not the means of obtaining the right state of mind. To take this posture is itself to have the right state of mind. There is no need to obtain some special state of mind.*

It is not even that the mind follows the body. It is that any idea of a mind separate from the body is a misunderstanding. We do not have to control the mind, we just have to learn to sit with it as it is. This does not mean that just because we sit in a good meditation posture, our mind will become calm and peaceful, but that when we adopt a posture we have a chance just to experience our mind as it is. Our posture offers the stability in sitting with our minds as they go through their routines of craving and aversion. The difference is that we are attentive to what the mind is doing.

To be attentive is to take care to notice. It is a receptive way of being with ourselves. This is not the same as being passive. There is nothing passive about the posture that forms the basis of our practice. We are attentive and alive to what is happening, but we are not trying to control it in the way that we usually try to control our experience. When something happens that we don't like, we usually try to deal with it in some way. We might try to distract ourselves, or to think it through, or we might just pretend that it didn't happen. We often do these things without very much awareness; we find ourselves reacting in one way or another. When we meditate, another option becomes available to us. It is available to us all the time, of course, but we are unaware of it. That option is to allow it to be as it is. The thing about allowing things to be as they are is that they never stay the same for very long anyway. Whether it is a itch on the face, sadness in the heart, or an uncomfortable thought of some kind, when you observe it closely you will notice that it changes. Left alone, it blinks into being and then transforms into something else.

This physical sense of ourselves allows us to watch our experience come and go; we do not collapse into the experience. So on the one hand we closely observe what is happening, on the other we keep a broader sense of awareness that includes our bodies, and the context we are in. There seems to be a problem here because we tend to confuse awareness with thinking. While it is very hard, though possible, to think of two things at once, awareness has a natural breadth that persists even when it has a focus. Think for a moment about driving a car or riding a bike. You are focused on the road in front of you, but if something happens on the periphery of your awareness you are likely to notice it. This is especially true when riding a bike, otherwise I would have been killed many years ago. When we sit to meditate, we are attentive to what is happening but we do not grasp at it and contract our awareness around it. It is true that if we become very absorbed in the object of our meditation, our sense of our body and its surroundings can diminish and become very subtle. Now if this happens, that's fine, I am not saying that you should try to stop it, however, this happens on the basis of having established a strong awareness within the body. If it happens without awareness of the body I think it is often a kind of alienated awareness.

So when we are meditating, the kind of awareness we try to cultivate is not solely dependent on this coming and going of our self-referential mental experience. It gains stability through awareness of our bodies and the context we are in. Another way of talking about this is to say that we cultivate big mind. Big mind is a feeling state that includes a sense of expansiveness. We all know the feeling of the mind going round in a circular fashion. Big mind means the sense of stepping back from this experience; part of the mind may be acting like a dog gnawing at a dry bone, but another part is aware of this happening and seeing it within a broader context. This broader context begins with our own bodies and extends into our environment: the earth beneath us, that sky above, and the breathing world all around us. Small mind, by contrast, is unable to open to the situation in which it finds itself. Instead, it contracts around itself, and experiences itself as the whole world.

Awareness of the body is the first stage of this process of allowing the mind to broaden, for the body, filled as it is with sensation and emotion, offers a rich underworld of experience. The idea of the underworld as a place of riches is found in classical mythology, as well as in the folklore of many cultures. In a sense, our bodies within are our own underworlds, not revealed to the world, a place to which we alone have access. On the level of feeling, we experience through the body, and it seems as if our bodies have a kind of memory. In particular, according to body-based therapies, traumatic events are stored in the body as armouring or tension. It is as if what cannot be held in consciousness is stuffed down into the body and repressed. It seems to me that our body holds our history, and once we pay attention to our bodies we enter a more intimate relationship with ourselves. The body can be said to correspond to the more unconscious aspects of our psyches. By paying kind attention to our bodies, our awareness is encouraged to explore our own underworld where the riches of our lives are to be found. Paradoxically, the underworld is also a place of connection, a place where we meet the universal aspects of our psyche, for it is teeming with a life that the ego is unable to appropriate. In the body and in the heart we open to the complex nature of our being, and through this experience of our multifarious nature we gain sympathy for others.

There is a well-known story in the Buddhist scriptures of a woman who, having lost her baby, comes to the Buddha carrying the corpse of the dead child, and pleads with the Buddha to help her.[10] The Buddha tells her that he can help her, but in order to do so he needs a mustard seed from a household free from the suffering of death. Of course, the woman is unable to find such a place, and during her frantic search she realizes the universal nature of her grief. This does not mean that the grief disappeared; anyone who has lost someone close to them will know that one is never completely free of loss and sadness. However, her feelings are transformed. Her grief has been made human. Rather than separating her from the world, it becomes a point of connection. Her grief provides her with an insight into the human condition.

The transformation of emotion through meditation is the recognition of the universal nature of emotion. That which is most intimately us, is also that which connects us with others. Part of a Mary Oliver poem called 'Wild Geese' comes to mind:

> *Tell me about despair, yours, and I will tell you mine.*
> *Meanwhile the world goes on.*
> *Meanwhile the sun and the clear pebbles of the rain*
> *are moving across the landscapes,...*

But the world does not go on despite your despair, it goes on with that despair woven into its very fabric. This is perhaps something of a cold comfort, or at least it appears to be so initially. The Buddha's offer of freedom from suffering is not an offer of a perfect world in which we live in perpetual bliss. He offers us the world as it is: a world in which we experience hope and despair, love and loss. This is a world filled with both remarkable wonders and terrible tragedies. It is the world as it is. The one thing we can change is the way we choose to pass through the world. In her poem, 'Kindness', another poet, Naomi Shihab Nye, writes,

> *Before you know kindness as the deepest thing inside,*
> *you must know sorrow as the other deepest thing.*
> *You must wake up with sorrow.*
> *You must speak to it till your voice*
> *catches the thread of all sorrows*
> *and you see the size of the cloth.*

What stands out for me in this verse are the words, 'You must speak to it till your voice catches the thread of all sorrows'. To speak to it implies something different from a passive acceptance; it encourages an active engagement with our hearts. We enter into a dialogue, but it is not a bargaining. There is no mustard seed. We speak in order to listen, in order that our voice changes from an isolated voice to one that is part of the human choir.

meditation: opening the heart

Sitting in your meditation posture, take time to get settled and comfortable, using your breath to help you become aware of your body. When you feel you have an overall sense of your body, bring your attention to your heart area. Again, use the breath to give you a sense of this area. Feel how the breath lifts the chest as you breathe in, cultivate a sense of the breath creating a sense of space around your heart, opening the area around your heart. Imagine that the space created by the breath is a space for the feelings in your heart.

When you are ready, introduce a sense of kindness towards yourself. Breathe gently into your heart area and wish yourself well. Once you feel a sense of goodwill towards yourself, bring to mind the fact that you have suffered. Have a sense that this kindness you feel extends to the suffering you have endured throughout your life. Your might recall a particular event when you felt pain or grief. Let the sense of suffering and the sense of kindness sit together in your heart. Breathe into your heart area and sit with the acknowledgement of your suffering. Just sit with the feeling rather than think about it. Invite the suffering into your heart. Feel free to let the sense of suffering go if it feels too much, but as far as possible stay with it, along with the feeling of goodwill towards yourself. Notice how it feels to sit with these ideas and feelings. Notice what happens in the body, how your heart feels.

After a while, let go of the awareness of your suffering and bring to mind an awareness of your capacity for joy. Perhaps remember a time when you felt joyful,

> *when everything was right in your life. Just as you allowed your heart to open to your suffering, let it open now to the joy. Sit for a while with a sense of your capacity for joy. Now try to have a sense of the relationship between your heart's capacity for suffering and for joy, a sense that both can be held in kindness, a sense of your heart being strong enough to hold this range of emotions. Have a sense of how these seemingly opposing experiences are related, both dependent on an open heart. Bring to mind how your suffering and your joy are the experiences of all human hearts, and that all people have the capacity for suffering and joy. Let your heart open to the world as it is, full of suffering, full of joy. Slowly let the mind relax, come back to the breath and a sense of kindness towards yourself. Then stop trying to do anything at all, and just sit for a while.*

I have written so far about what we might call the more difficult side of the emotions we might encounter in meditation, but that is just one side of the story. The other side is the joy, bliss, and happiness that can arise during meditation. Just as our difficult emotions have corresponding physical feelings in the body, so our positive emotions can also be felt in the body. Just as we can work directly through the body to release negative emotions, so we can use the body to encourage positive aspects of our experience. In a way, we do the same thing whatever the emotion might be; we try to open up around it. We do not grasp at our experience, as we tend to do when something feels good. Buddhism teaches us that craving and aversion are two sides of the same coin. Both are reactions of the ego and both tighten rather then open up our sense of ourselves. Our response to a feeling such as joy should be just to sit with it, and open the mind and the body around it. When the body is aligned and relaxed, these feelings find a natural home. Indeed, the feeling of aliveness that we encourage through paying kind attention to our bodies will allow these positive feelings to emerge. When we learn to meditate with the body, these feelings are close at hand.

These emotions, while welcome, can also present a problem. I have found over many years of teaching meditation that many of us have problems accepting what feels good in our practice, and indeed in our lives. In the first stage of the traditional Buddhist practice called the loving-kindness meditation, we encourage a sense of love for ourselves. This sounds as though it should be an enjoyable thing, but many people find it distressing, for many of us feel we don't deserve unconditional love from ourselves, we feel unworthy, we feel we are not good enough, or that it is self-indulgent to encourage such feelings. I am not going to try to explain this in any detail. There are enough self-help books out there that offer explanations and suggest answers to a problem that seems to be particularly prevalent in western culture. I think it has something to do with our Christian heritage, and also, of course, with our individual backgrounds, but I don't think we have to unravel our cultural and family backgrounds to accept self-love; there is a more direct approach that we can take through meditation. This is not to say that we might not need other forms of assistance. Meditation is not a magic bullet, but it can play an important part in learning to love and care for ourselves.

In sitting with my own experience, I have myself noticed the tendency I mentioned earlier of trying to bargain with myself. The thinking mind is very fond of this sort of thing. In saying this, I am reminded of those folk stories in which someone is given three wishes – it always seems to be three – and they end up in a worse situation than when they started. These tales seem to be trying to show us that although we wish to be different from who we are, this only leads us further away from ourselves.

Think for a minute of a situation in which you are in the company of a close friend who is in a bad way. Perhaps their lover has recently left them; anyway, they are quite distressed. What is your response in that type of situation? Do you pat them on the back and tell them there are plenty more fish in the sea? You have probably found that this isn't helpful. In these situations people just want you to be with them. There really isn't anything you can do to make it all right, but you can be with them and be kind and attentive. You can let them speak, to say what they need to say, to cry. You don't have to try to put things right. In sitting with people who are dying, I have found that just to be as fully present as you can with another person can be an act of love. When you are able to let go of wanting to make things better, and accept the situation as it is, then intimacy can open up. The same thing can happen with ourselves when we meditate. If we let go of bargaining and wanting to be different, a sense of love towards ourselves can develop based on the situation as it is. There is a poem from the Shin Buddhist tradition that expresses this kind of radical acceptance.

You, as you are, you're just right.
Your face, body, name, surname,
For you, they are just right.

Whether poor or rich,
Your parents, your children,
    your daughter-in-law, your grandchildren,
They are all, for you, just right.

Happiness, unhappiness, joy and even sorrow.
For you, they are just right.

The life that you have trod is neither good nor bad,
For you, it is just right.

Whether you go to hell or to the Pure Land,
Wherever you go is just right.

Nothing to boast about, nothing to feel bad about,
Nothing above, nothing below.
Even the day and month that you die,
Even they are just right.

Life in which you walk together with Amida,
There's no way that it can't be just right.

When you receive your life as just right,
Then a deep and profound trust begins to open up.

Amida is a archetypal figure, a Bodhisattva, who represents infinite light and love. This poem presents a challenge to open up to one's life as it is in each moment. Meditation offers us an opportunity to do this simply and directly. We sit with what is happening in the moment. In this sense, meditation takes a certain kind of courage. The word 'courage' is related to the French word for 'heart', and we still say 'to take heart', so we can think of meditation as taking heart. By 'heart' I mean both the emotional side of our experience and our core beliefs and values. Some people are lucky enough to feel they are driven by some need, such as to be an artist, which they cannot help but act upon, but for many, our fate is hidden, overlaid by the expectations of other people or just the pressures of daily life. When we meditate in an open and receptive way we give these hidden parts of ourselves a chance to come more fully into awareness. I am not encouraging you to daydream when you meditate, but I am saying that the psychic space that meditation creates does allow what is deepest in ourselves to rise to the surface of our minds. I always try to remember to tell people new to meditation that it is quite a dangerous thing to take up. It is dangerous because it has the power to bring to the fore aspirations that have been buried under the life one has led, to reveal the as yet unlived life, and this can create conflict. It may mean that one becomes confronted with difficult choices as the desire to lead a more meaningful life is reconnected with and develops. This is a good thing, of course, but it is not always comfortable.

Socrates is reputed to have said that 'the unexamined life is not worth living'. I think he meant that a life in which we do not look deeply inside to find ourselves is an unlived life. It may be that we have no particular mission in life, but nevertheless I feel we all have a certain calling. It is not necessarily a calling to do something special in the world, but a calling toward authenticity, to be as fully ourselves as we are able. In the celebrity-obsessed culture in which we find ourselves, it is all too easy to think that fame is the only mark of a successful life, but of course our own sense of a life lived well depends not on outside validation but an inner sense of being fully ourselves, developing our innate capacity to experience and express love and kindness.

the body and the loving-kindness meditation

One of the most popular meditations in the Buddhist tradition is called the loving-kindness meditation, though it seems to be a problematic meditation for many people. This is largely because there is a gap between what we 'think' should happen in the meditation and our actual experience of doing it. It is easy to have the expectation that if we are doing the meditation correctly we should experience a flood of love, when in reality we find that the practice leaves us numb, or we struggle with distraction and restlessness. This leaves us feeling bad about ourselves, which is of course quite the opposite from what is intended. The first thing is to try the meditation with a spirit of inquiry, so the focus of the practice becomes a sense of interest in what our experience actually is. This spirit of taking an interest is vital. Each time we sit for meditation we should be open to something quite new. This is sometimes known as 'beginner's mind', which means we do not prejudge ourselves. The shift of focus from wanting a particular result to just taking a kind interest in what is really happening means that we remove the pressure of wanting a 'good' meditation.

In the loving-kindness meditation we develop an intention to promote a feeling of loving-kindness. We often have to start with the idea of kindness while we are not actually in touch with those feelings. So we notice what it feels like to bring such an idea to mind, we take a kindly interest in our reaction. This 'idea' might be a directed thought such as 'may I care deeply for myself', or it might take the form of an image or even a imagined bodily feeling, such as a sense of warmth or openness around the heart. In this way we introduce a suggestion of love, and then we take care to notice what happens, how we respond to that suggestion. We do not try to impose the feeling on ourselves, we cannot force ourselves to feel loving-kindness. All we can do is to try to approach the practice with kindness. That is to say, the atmosphere in which we undertake the practice should be one of loving-kindness. This means that we do our best to treat whatever happens, even if it seems to be contradictory to what we think should happen, with kindness.

Kindness in this sense is very close to simply taking a genuine interest in our experience. If, for instance, we introduce the idea of feeling loving-kindness towards ourselves, and we notice that our reaction is one of self-hatred, that we do not deserve to be loved, we don't compound that reaction, we don't go on to think how bad we are that we can't feel kindness towards ourselves. Instead, we apply kindness to that reaction. Think how you would like to respond to a child's expression of self-hatred. What would you do? What emotion would that initiate in you? Imagine your own child expressing self-loathing. Surely tenderness would fill your heart, you would reach out to your child with love. Many of our feelings towards ourselves are regressive, based on past experience, based on the lack of tenderness and love being available when we needed them. Every time you do this meditation is an opportunity to open your heart to yourself. In order for this to be possible, you have to be prepared to sit with the pain in a loving and interested way. It is not easy, but it is a chance for healing to take place. When we open to what is there, the possibility of change opens up.

This opening to our experience is based not so much in the rational mind. The rational mind will tend to avoid, will seek to distract us, to protect us by moving away from our direct experience, particularly if that experience is painful. I have talked of the body as representing the unconscious; what is repressed is held in the body. When you feel the mind moving away, closing down to your experience, try to use that direct experience of your physical body to stay with what is happening. Feel the numbness, and breathe into the hurt. Open the body around your heart. Think of loving-kindness as a willingness to abide with what is there in your heart. Don't try to rationalize your experience away; notice what the rational mind does: the arguments, the fabrication. Watch it with kindness, meet it with kindness, gently telling yourself to stay with the feeling. What does it really feel like on the level of sensation? Work with the constriction around the heart, meet yourself in the pain. If we try to superimpose loving-kindness over of our felt experience, we push the hurt, the grief, and the pain further down. There is no loving-kindness without the frank acknowledgement of what is really there in our hearts. None of us gets through life without suffering hurt, rejection, and grief. These are the feelings that need to be met with interested and kindness, for although they initially seem to isolate us from others, they are in fact points of true connection. Remember the story about the woman who lost her only child; her search for a mustard seed brought her to a new understanding of the universal nature of suffering and a new level of compassion that embraced her along with all of humanity.

If you are one of the many people who have difficulty making a emotional connection with this practice, I suggest you try seeing that practice in terms of an inquiry into your own heart rather than an attempt to 'generate' loving-kindness. Furthermore, see the practice as abiding with your response and don't feel you have to be busy within it. You should establish a sense of connection with your body and breath and maintain this throughout the meditation, returning to that connection whenever you get distracted. There are many ways of undertaking this meditation, and you should feel free to experiment and find an approach that works for you, although on the whole it is best to keep it simple. What follows is a guided meditation that I hope you will find useful.

meditation: loving-kindness using the body and the breath

Sitting in your meditation posture, take whatever time you need to get comfortable and let the body settle.

Begin by listening to the world around you, let whatever you hear remind you that you are in the world and that this practice is performed within the context of the world and for the world as well as yourself. Do not strain to hear, just notice whatever sounds there are, and how they naturally enter your awareness and fall away. As you listen, let your face start to relax and soften. Notice how your face feels. Imagine your face letting go around the eyes and jaw. Notice what your face feels like, as if you are listening to your face. Your face is what you show to the world, and we sometimes feel obliged to put on a brave face, but see if you can just let your face express your heart. Breathe your face, letting it soften on your out-breath. Feel how sensitive your face is, how it holds your character and history. Let your face speak to you. From the face, slowly move through the rest of your body, using your breath to support this awareness. Use your imagination. For example, imagine your spine, alive, made up not just of bone but of soft tissue, nerves, and fluid. Breathe into the different areas of your body; for example, breathing in, be aware of the pelvis, breathing out, be aware of the pelvis. If any images of particular feelings, emotions, or thoughts related to this kind listening to your body arise, be aware of them. Try not to elaborate on them with the rational mind, just let the image or feeling be there until it fades away. As you become aware of different areas of your body, encourage a sense of appreciation for them, recognizing how they fundamentally enrich your life. I find the hands particularly good in this respect.

If parts of your body feel numb, breathe a warm kind breath into them. Don't force them to respond, just listen to them and be open to whatever arises. Take your time, seeing this as an act of loving-kindness towards your body. Pay particular attention to your belly and the area around your heart, approaching it receptively, letting your body say what it wants to say, rather than trying to force awareness into it or demanding a response. Do not interrogate the body, but abide with it and let it sing its songs. The body might speak to us both directly, through sensations, and through images. Perhaps your hands feel like birds, your belly like an oven, your heart like a stone. Be sensitive to the language, accept the image or the thought, however outlandish it might be. If you find images arising, let them speak to you directly rather than try to interpret them.

When you feel ready, introduce the idea of loving-kindness with a simple phrase that resonates with you. See if you can let it come to you as from the heart. Imagine your heart speaking directly. Use your breath to open up a sense of space around your heart and listen to the longing that enters that space. If nothing comes, suggest a phrase to your heart, such as 'may I care deeply for myself,' 'may I love myself as I am in this moment.' Watch and listen to your body, imagine what loving-kindness feels like in your body. Most importantly, treat yourself with kindness.

In the other stages of the meditation,[9] try to maintain a sense of your body. One thing I often do is just imagine someone else breathing as I breathe. So the breath becomes a link. As you breathe in, think of them breathing in, as you breathe out, think of them breathing out. Imagine the breath opening their heart as it opens yours, imagine the breath bringing life into their body as it brings life into yours. In this way, we keep the practice simple and direct, we encourage the feeling of interconnection, an awareness of the life-force that we share with all beings. Let go of any idea of having to 'produce' loving-kindness and pump it out, be content just to breathe with it.

There is no 'right' way of doing this meditation, but it is better to understand it in terms of an inquiry into your heart, rather than an exercise in which you manufacture love and then send it out into the world to help others. This seems a bit too much for most of us, and even has the danger of making us feel we are in some sense better than those poor people who are so in need of our loving-kindness.

The rather paradoxical aspect of the loving-kindness meditation, which is, after all, concerned with our emotions, is that, in many people, it provokes too much thought, so we should avoid making up stories, and just keep to very simple direct thoughts, all the time remaining aware of the body, particularly around the heart and the belly.

6

the body and insight

At the core of the Buddha's teachings lies the idea that it is possible for all human beings to achieve insight into their true nature and the nature of reality, and that this achieving of insight is what allows people to overcome the experience of dissatisfaction that dominates their lives. Although insight might arise at any time, meditation is the most effective means of encouraging this.

The Buddhist idea of insight is really very simple. It means seeing ourselves as we are and the world as it is. This 'seeing' does not take place through the physical eye but through direct experience of ourselves and the world. This means that we bring ourselves into a sympathetic relationship with how things really are, rather than wanting the world to conform to our desires. It is this gap between how things are and our egoistic expectations of how things should be that causes of so much of our suffering. Insight is not a metaphysical problem; there is no secret world to be discovered, or mystery to be penetrated. The world reveals itself to us as it is, but our ignorance and delusion prevents our seeing it. Insight, as the term implies, means seeing inside. It reveals that we are not separate from the world, that the qualities apparent all around us in the world also apply to us. According to Buddhism, reality has three marks, or *lakshanas*. Stated in the negative, these are impermanence, insubstantiality, and unsatisfactoriness. These could equally be seen in positive terms; we could say that the world is dynamic, alive, and full of beauty. Behind these marks is not their negative or positive attributes, which are dependent on the way that we, as subjects, view them, but the 'is-ness' of the world. What is being asked of us is that we see that nothing is fixed, everything is subject to change, and that nothing is totally discrete from everything else. Most importantly, this insight needs to be directly experienced in relation to ourselves. It is therefore often expressed as the overcoming of the experience of the self as something that is permanent and fixed, and therefore different from the world around us.

Buddhism does not claim that we do not have a feeling of selfhood. Indeed it is this feeling that we are a subject that seems to mark out humans from most other living things. We are human because we feel there is an agency behind our feelings and thoughts. This is our experience, and saying that it is not so makes very little difference to this experience. So it is clear that Buddhist insight is something quite different from knowing in the normal sense of that term. If anything is going to change, it is on a different level of knowing that it needs to change. Some of the confusion that arises with this topic of 'no self' can be clarified by asking how we actually experience our 'self' on a moment-to-moment basis. What I think we will find is that our sense of self is what we might call a background feeling. For example, as we are reading these words, there is also a sense that 'we' are reading. That is to say, there is some background feeling behind the complex activity of reading, which although subtle is sufficient to give us a feeling that it is 'us' reading.

In his book, *The Feeling of What Happens*, Antonio Damasio deals with the biological underpinning of consciousness, and emphasizes the importance of bodily feelings and emotions in the formation of the feeling we have of being ourselves, pointing out that it is a feeling rather than an idea that gives us a sense of self. So if our sense of self is feeling based, rather than cognitive, it means that if we wish to change the way we experience ourselves we have to take notice of our feelings and emotions. This perhaps helps us to see why just knowing that there is no basis for seeing the self as fixed and unchanging is of little help in the practical matter of changing our experience and behaviour in the world, because it is our feelings, not our ideas, that largely determine the way we are. The more attached we are to this feeling of self, the more likely we are to react to anything that threatens it. Think of a time when you were upset with someone. Behind the way we react to others there is often a feeling that we have been hurt or frustrated in some way. But what is this 'we' that has been hurt or frustrated?

This notion that the self is a feeling, rather than an idea, is also reflected in the traditional list of the three 'poisons' that create the volitional agency of the ego. These are greed, hatred, and delusion. The third, which sounds as though it could relate to the rational mind, is much more than that. It refers to our basic experience of ourselves. It is not possible to think ourselves free from delusion; that is to overestimate the power of the rational mind. When it comes to the Buddhist idea of insight, the rational mind alone is of limited use. This is partly because we rarely experience our delusion directly. Instead, it is veiled by the very physical emotional complex of greed and hatred, these most primal and typical motivators of human behaviour. Somehow our delusion has to be accessed through these gatekeepers. Until this is achieved, it is extremely difficult to work directly with our delusion. It is hard to step out of a delusional system because we can only act from a deluded state. Although we find examples of dramatic and sudden breakthroughs within the Buddhist scriptures – in one well-known story[11] a mass murderer gains this insight after a short exchange with the Buddha – we cannot make this happen, and a more realistic approach is to work with our greed and hatred which are the emotional supports of our delusion.

Delusion is directly related to our feeling of self; as such it is also what we might broadly call a feeling. This is not to say that our delusion doesn't have a cognitive component, but that this component is founded on sensational and emotional experience, which can be directly felt in the body. Delusion is not just an idea; we become aware of it mostly as feeling. Delusion is found in the body as feeling. Take an example such as anger. We feel anger, and of course we also have angry thoughts, but these are defined by the feeling behind them. What often happens, however, is that we lose touch with the bodily experience, and we are left with our ingrained ways of thinking about the world separate from the physical experience of anger that gave rise to them. The words we find in the Buddhist scriptures relating to the cause of delusion, along with expressions of greed such as thirst, craving, grasping, all have a very visceral sense, indicating that our delusion is not merely intellectual misunderstanding. They relate as much, if not more, to the body as to the rational mind.

I hope this does not sound too complicated, but it is important to understand it, as it is vital to why the body is so important in relation to meditation. Our relationship to our bodily feelings forms the foundation for the delusion that prevents us entering a full relationship with our true nature and the world of which we are part. Our sense or feeling of the self has its origins in the relationship between our awareness and bodily experience.

I once found myself in a lot of discomfort during an intensive meditation retreat. I couldn't sit still. The idea of another meditation session filled me with dread. I remember sitting down and thinking to myself I could either spend the next forty minutes squirming in discomfort, or I could just sit with whatever was going on. I decided just to sit with the discomfort. In the course of that meditation, something fundamental shifted in my understanding of meditation. I realized I could sit with my discomfort, indeed I could use the sensations as aids to meditation rather than seeing them as hindrances. For me, the key to doing this was very simple and something that I knew very well in theory: it was just to bide with them in a kindly way, to stop resisting them and accept them on their own level, that is, as pure sensation.

This was not the first time I had done this, but this time something else happened. I started to experience the thoughts that went along with the discomfort as simply another level of sensation. This might not sound anything special, indeed it is not, but it completely changed my relationship with my meditation experience. Furthermore, it has largely stayed with me. For the first time, I was able to experience the sensations that I was interpreting as pain as mere sensations. I need to add an important note here. If you really are in pain, particularly in vulnerable parts of the body such as the knees, do not try to sit through it. Move. There is a qualitative difference between real pain, which indicates that you are damaging your body, and the everyday discomfort that we all sometimes feel in meditation. The kind of restlessness and discomfort I was experiencing had more to do with hitting a level of resistance. So I somehow managed to stop adding to the sensations I felt, and by taking an interest in them I started to experience them in a way that helped me to feel absorbed.

This was followed by an extension of this same principle to mental sensations. All our experience is mental, in the sense that it is experienced by our minds, but an itch is normally regarded as being quite different from an idea. An itch is something that is happening to us, and a thought is something that we are doing. However, in meditation we realize that most of what goes on, on the level of thought, is just happening. All that chatter arises in the mind unbidden, and we have, it seems, little more control over it than the physical sensations that arise in the body. This being the case, there is no particular reason why we should treat them differently. We need to stop attaching the idea of a self to them.

I am reminded of a routine the black comic Richard Prior used to perform. He began by demonstrating a white man walking through the jungle. He walks tentatively along and nearly treads on a snake. Completely freaked out, he screams and does a little uncoordinated dance. Then he demonstrates a black man, who calmly steps over the snake and cooly says, 'snake', and walks on as before. Well you have to see it, but nevertheless it is a rather appropriate analogy of what happens in meditation, for we will encounter snakes of all kinds. It is our reaction to them that is important. We should not try to avoid such encounters by keeping to safe and familiar paths, which would involve trying to control our experience. We should be attentive and notice, but we don't have to make a fuss. How can we do this? As I have said already, the stability is sought in the posture: we sit as though we mean business. Through our posture we develop confidence, we employ our imagination to be aware of our body on the level of sensation. Such

awareness supports a moment-to-moment awareness based on our direct experience of aliveness. This
breadth of awareness stops us falling into an exclusively mental experience in which we are liable to get
caught in anxiety or fantasy.

I have often thought it appropriate to talk metaphori-
cally of the body as the unconscious. By this I mean
that the body is the storehouse, the hill in which the
treasure is hidden. It is the place of the emotions and
where we keep our hearts. When we sit, there should
be a sense of taking care of, and with, the body. Sometimes the idea of being mindful is expressed as 'abiding with'. I like that very much. 'Abide' comes to us
from a Gothic root meaning to wait, so it has the suggestion of waiting with. We wait with the body. To
wait suggests we have stopped. To abide with the
body is to wait with, having stopped our normal chat-
tering. But to abide is more than to wait. It certainly
does not involve the finger-tapping sort of waiting,
for it also implies a physical closeness. The image of
the mind abiding with the breath and the body suggests a 'being in'. In this sense it provokes a coming
home, the self coming home. In a sense it is a return to
Eden, which is the great Christian symbol of what we
might now call the unconscious.

Coming back to the body has all the mythology of
coming home. James Hillman comments on returning
to the family house in his essay 'Mythology as
Family'. It is such a wonderful piece that I will quote it
at length.

> *The debilitating energy loss strikes everyone alike as if a communal power outage. Everyone caught in repeating, and resisting, old patterns. Nothing changed, after all these years! No one can get out even for a walk to break the spell, the whole family sinking deeper into the upholstery (and the television has little to do with it and may even be, in such moments, the household god who saves). These moments attest to the capacity of family for sharing – French anthropology used to speak of a participation mystique – in a common soul or psychic state, and for containing the regressive needs of the soul. No one is at fault, no one is kicked out, and no one can be helped. In the paralysis lies the profoundest source of acceptance. Grandpa can go on grumbling, brother attacking the administration, sister introvertly attending her exacerbating eczema, and mother go on covering up with solicitous busyness. Everyone goes down the drain because family love allows family pathology, an immense tolerance for the hopeless shadow in each, the shadow that we each carry as permanent part of our baggage and that we unpack when we go back home.*[12]

Coming back home is a little like coming back to the body. At least, it feels like that at times. Here the relationship between posture and awareness is critical, as it is too easy to sink into the upholstery or watch the television. It is our posture that prevents us sinking without trace. Just as our families hold our history and we theirs, so, in a sense, do our bodies. When people try to be aware of their bodies they often feel very tired. Alternatively, they turn up the internal television. Our posture saves us because it allows us to abide. We need to be alert to our tendency to be drawn into a narrative version of our mental experience. This in no way excludes imagination, but, as Hillman would say, we stay with the image. We abide with it, we try not to interrogate it. We listen to it, and we encourage a sense that it happens within the breath-body. The breath allows the body to express itself. Linking the breath and the body is to be aware of the breath of the body. We should not separate them. It would be a mistake to think that we drop one level of awareness when we take up the next. We do not drop the awareness of the breath for the body, or the body for emotion, emotion for thought. Instead, they are the environment in which that awareness is happening. The practice is *earthed* through the body. The body connects with the earth and the world. To sit is to touch the earth, to abide with the earth. To breathe is to become aware of being in a breathing world. Here we have a confident ground for the practice. We have called the earth goddess. We have earth, sky, and breathing world to support us. We have our families and our history. We abide with this as an act of faith. The internationally renowned potter Shoji Hamada comments in his book, *The Unknown Craftsman*,

> If a kiln is small, I might be able to control it completely, that is to say, my own self can become a controller, a master of the kiln. But man's own self is but a small thing after all. When I work at the large kiln, the power of my own self becomes so feeble that it cannot control it adequately. It means that for the

large kiln, the power that is beyond me is necessary.
Without the mercy for such an invisible power I
cannot get good pieces. One of the reasons why I
wanted to have a large kiln is because I want to be a
potter, if I may, who works more in grace than in his
own power. You know nearly all the best pots were
done in a huge kiln.[13]

Hamada's reflection on working as a craftsman reminds me of alchemy, which is often referred to as a
craft. Within craft there is repetition. Meditation is
also a craft. It is like making bread. We trust in a
household god and yeast. In meditation, our bodies
are the kiln. When we work with a small mind we can
perhaps control it, with big mind we abide. We give it
our attention as best we can and keep our fingers
crossed. Any attempt to control the situation is a bit
like repeatedly opening the oven door to see if the
bread has started to rise. The alchemist repeats and
repeats, knowing that as he or she changes the subject, so must the object change. The work is the life.
When we sit to meditate we should understand that
this is a chance to be fully ourselves, that is, to let the
whole of ourselves be there; not just the part that
would be the master of the situation, but all of us.

principles of bodywork in meditation
establishing the ground
People often think of meditation as something that
happens in our heads, but if this is our view of meditation we deny ourselves the ground that can give
stability and strength to our practice. Meditation
always takes place somewhere, at a particular time
and place. When we sit, we sit on the earth with the

sky above us. We sit indoors or outside. We should be aware of the particular context in which we sit to meditate, and allow that context to support our practice. When we are fortunate enough to meditate with others, we should be aware of them and allow the collective nature of the practice to support us. In meditation, we are ultimately concerned with overcoming the dualism of self and other. When meditation is understood as something that just goes on in our head, we reinforce that sense of dualism. Alternatively, we can be receptive to the physical and imaginative context in which we practise, and by doing so establish a sense of being grounded. This includes taking care even before you sit down. I have often seen people come into the meditation room chatting to one another – I have done it myself – then picking up the mat and cushions and throwing them carelessly on the ground. The alternative is to introduce mindfulness. You can take care with the mat and cushions. They can be placed with a sense of purpose. You are preparing your seat, and the way you do that will affect your experience. Your meditation does not have to wait for the starting bell, it can start with the way you remove and arrange your shoes, how you walk into the room, how you make your seat, how you place your body.

People often think that we meditate to become mindful or to encourage loving-kindness, but this is the wrong way to understand it. Meditation is an opportunity to express qualities of awareness and kindness. Of course, our lives constantly present such opportunities, but if we are unable to do so in our approach to meditation, how likely is it that we will be able to do so in the rest of our lives?

So notice and take care what you are doing when you prepare for meditation. In this way you are already expressing qualities of awareness and kindness. This is why we sometimes do little rituals before we meditate. We might light a candle because this brings us into the present and prepares us. In some Zen traditions, the student is taught to bow in various directions after entering the zendo, or meditation hall. They are also taught to position their mat carefully, smoothing out any wrinkles, and then to take care centring the cushion on the mat, so that by the time they actually sit down they are already in a state of mindfulness. The important point is that we bring mindfulness and kindness to the practice. Rather than seeing meditation as an activity that produces these qualities, we see it as an expression of the qualities inherent in ourselves.

Meditation is also an act of imagination, meaning the ability to employ our awareness in a particular way. This sort of imagination should not be confused with fantasy. We use our imaginative ability to remember the world, the earth and the sky and the life all around us. In this way we allow the world to support us. We imagine the earth beneath us and notice that it supports us unconditionally in that moment. We have taken our place with care and we allow ourselves to imagine that the world is on our side, for we are part of that world, it is in us and all around us. So we are aware of the context in which we meditate and encourage a sense of reverence for the world that is our home.

Along with the world, the other context to notice is the body. Our bodies are the 'we' manifestation of the world. The body is naturally attuned to the wider world, for it has come from that world, so we can look at this process of grounding the practice as simply listening to our bodies: we pay attention to them, receptively allowing them to tell their story, to sing their song.

embodying awareness
By this process of paying attention to our bodies, and noticing sensations, feelings, and emotions as they arise, we encourage our natural awareness of the body. We are aware through and in our bodies rather than feeling that our awareness is just in our heads. In this way, we pay attention to our direct experience rather than just our thoughts. The body is always full of sensation – for example, our buttocks, legs, and feet are full of the sensations of contact with the floor. These feelings of contact are constantly changing and are always available to us. In addition, the face is very sensitive to the air around it, and full of changing sensations.

By noticing our bodies on this level of sensation, our awareness is drawn into the body and helps us to un-lock the mind from its habitual thoughts and con-cerns. Beginning with these obvious sensations, we can then become aware how other areas of the body feel. The belly and the area around the heart are par-ticularly important, as these regions tend to be where feeling and emotion come together. We might use our breath to help us bring awareness into these areas. It is still mainly a matter of just being receptive and then aware of what arises when the attention is focused in these areas of the body. By just noticing what our bodies feel like, we start to gain an intuitive sense of the interrelationship between sensation, emotion, and thought. Our awareness begins to be embodied.

If, for instance, you pay attention to your belly, you might notice a tightness or a feeling of unease. Staying with that feeling, certain thoughts or images might come to mind. If this happens, be aware of them but also try to stay aware of the area of the body that is related to them coming to mind. In this way, thoughts or images are felt in the body. You might be tempted to move awareness from the body, and get caught up in the thought or the image, which then becomes disembodied and takes on a life of its own, moving towards abstraction and rationalization. To counter this tendency, breathe into the area and remain aware of the sensational experience. This will get easier the more you do it. After a while, you will be able to maintain attention on your body when thoughts and images arise.

anchoring the practice

We all get distracted when we meditate. Our thoughts depart from our direct experience of the object of our attention. When this happens, bring the mind back to the body, first re-establishing mindfulness of your direct experience. For example, if you are focusing on your breathing and you realize that your attention has drifted, do not try to force it back. First, bring it back to the basic elements of the situation. Re-establish the ground of the meditation and then an awareness of your body, posture, and the sensations in the body. Then bring back a sense of your breath. This does not have to take long. Indeed, it can all happen in a few seconds once you have become used to working in this way. If you don't do this, the mind will tend to distraction again. The practice of using the ground and your body as a way of anchoring your meditation will greatly help to reduce the distraction and is well worth spending time on. Like all things in meditation, this is a matter of feeling. While sometimes it might take only a few seconds to re-establish the ground and embodied feeling to the practice, at other times most of the meditation will be taken up with it. This is time well spent, for if these foundations are not in place, whatever else you do will lack depth and be more akin to day-dreaming than meditation.

The awareness and kindness that we aim to develop in meditation are clearly qualities that are potentially present at all times. Sometimes, however, it is easy to forget about them as soon as we rise from the cushion. One of the ways that we can start to bring the awareness that we experience in meditation into other areas of our lives is through mindful walking. Walking meditation can be a very useful practice, and for some people it is more effective than sitting meditation, as the physical activity of walking gives the mind a constant stream of clear sensations to engage with. There are many forms of walking meditation. My personal favourite comes from the Zen tradition, and it is a form that links the breathing to the steps we take. I will describe it as it was taught to me, but you may wish to do it a little differently.

meditation: walking meditation

> Start by just standing still and becoming aware of the pattern of your breathing. Just breathe naturally. Now on the in-breath slowly lift your right foot, take a small step about the length of your foot, and then carefully place the foot down, toes first, breathing out as you do so. Just take one small step with each cycle of the breath. Placing the toes first makes it a little easier to balance, but it is also counterintuitive and requires attention. One you are used to taking the steps, try not to look down at your feet, and maintain an upright posture. I have found this a very good way to become mindful. Linking each step to the breath means that you really have to pay attention. It is rather slow, so you also get the physical sensation of slowing down, which I like.

Some people find this slow walking frustrating. If you do, that might be a good reason to stick with it. For any form of walking meditation to be effective, it should be continued for a while. I do this slow walking for about forty minutes at a time.

If you are doing this in a public place you might want to walk more normally, but this can also be effective. Find a physical focus for the practice. Perhaps the best focus is the feet, making and breaking contact with the ground. The sensations in the feet should be quite distinct, so it is fairly easy to stay with them. While there is this focus, you can also be aware of the rest of the body. In particular, make sure your shoulders are relaxed, cultivate a sense of what the body feels like moving through space, let the face soften and let yourself enjoy walking. As with sitting meditation, if the mind wanders, bring it gently back to your direct experience of walking. Try to keep your steps even and your pace consistent, and let the steady rhythm of your walking help relax your body.

You might also try introducing a sense of loving-kindness into a walking meditation. You can do this by having the idea of placing the feet with a sense of care. Using your imagination, you might also encourage a sense of the earth on which you tread, playing with the notion that the way you carefully and lovingly place your feet is an act of acknowledgement, even reverence, towards the earth. This is more a matter of feeling than thinking, but of course thought can be used to stimulate feeling just as feeling stimulates thought. Walking meditation can be a very good way to become more mindful, and some people find it more engaging than sitting. Regular practice will also spill over into your experience of walking at other times. You will become more aware of your bodily movements in general, and this helps you to stay centred as you go about your daily life.

7

world, body, and soul

In this concluding chapter I want to say a little about the relationship between our bodies and the world in which we live. I want to suggest that our bodies and minds, although we experience them as somehow separate, are in fact just part of the world. In a way, this is obvious, but it is not our normal experience of being in the world. Meditation is important because it offers us a direct means of breaking down the sense of separation and isolation that causes us, individually and collectively, so much pain and suffering. Throughout this book I have suggested that meditation should be understood as a means of becoming more embodied, and that this can be achieved by paying kind attention to our felt experience, especially within our bodies.

If we are embodied, we are also 'emworlded', that is, we are part of the world in which we live. This is one of the main insights of many spiritual traditions, and one that modern science is recently coming to appreciate through its theories on emergence, which suggest not only that the organism adapts to its environment, but that the environment adapts to the organism. They are in a constant and dynamic relationship with each other, they co-emerge. For example, take the ability of bees to see the colour of flowers. It turns out that flowers developed colour at the same time that bees developed the ability to see it. There would be no point in flowers displaying themselves in that way if there were no bees to see them, and no point in bees seeing in that way if there were no coloured flowers to see. Biologists are now talking about the co- emergence of the environment and particular organisms, their point being that there is not so much an environment out there that we respond to, but that we are part of that environment. Richard Lewontin puts it as follows.

> *The organism and the environment are not actually separately determined. The environment is not a structure imposed on living beings from the outside but is in fact a creation of those beings. The environment is not an autonomous process but a reflection of the biology of the species. Just as there is no organism without an environment, so there is no environment without an organism.*[14]

This is, of course, not a new idea, but a very old one, re-expressed in the language of modern science. It is a central teaching of Buddhism that the seeming separateness of things is a delusion. The teaching of Indra's Net is a well known metaphor for this: we are asked to imagine that reality is like a vast net of jewels, and that every jewel is reflected in every other jewel. If modern science and Buddhism are right, the implications are immense. If we felt this intimate sense of being in and of the world, our lives would be transformed. It is hard to see how we are going to have the courage to face up to the global problems that now confront us, unless there is such a fundamental change in the way we understand our place in the world. But the teaching of Indra's Net also offers us hope, because it implies that we can influence the world around us. More than that, it teaches us that our way of being in the world affects the world, just as the world affects us.

When we sit to meditate, we often go into the practice with a very different perception of our relationship to the world and the way things really are. We feel that there is us, and then there is everything else, the world. Far from feeling part of that world – that it supports us and is on our side, we might say – we feel the world is a rather hostile place. We do not feel at home in the world but out of place. From the point of view of the ego, the world is often hostile, it frustrates us, it is never quite as we would like it. By shifting our focus from what is going on in our heads to just noticing how things are at that moment, we might discover that we feel rather different about the world and ourselves. When we come home to our bodies on the level of direct experience, we also come home to the world. If we don't feel we belong in our bodies, how are we to feel that we belong in the world, which is co-emergent with them?

When people sit to meditate, they often do so in a particular place and at a particular time: they meditate with the world. Far from understanding meditation as a means of somehow removing ourselves from the world, and getting into our own private space that has little to do with the real world, we can meditate in a way that allows us to feel supported by the world. To do this we use our imagination. We imagine what is outside, and its relationship to us.

meditation: being in the world

Take your time getting comfortable. Feel the earth beneath you. Let it support you. Think of the earth extending in all directions beneath you. Feel the energy of the living earth, being aware of the life all around you. Feel the energy inside your body. Have a sense that the energy inside and outside your body is the same energy, the energy of life. Use awareness of your breath to help you feel the connection between the universe inside you and the universe outside you. Imagine that you are breathing through the whole surface of your skin, feel the porosity of your skin, encouraging a sense that your skin is not what separates you from the whole world – you inside, the world outside – but that the skin is porous, and as you breathe you come into the world and the world comes into you. Maintain a sense of the earth spreading out beneath you.

Now, as you breathe out, start to imagine not only your breath going out into the world but also your awareness. First, just imagine the awareness moving a few inches out all around you, as if your mind is moving out into the world with your breath. Still imagine that you are breathing out through the whole of your skin, so your mind is very slowly moving out all around you. Don't try to force your awareness, just imagine it is

> *slowly and gently expanding out from your body along with the breath, not so much thinking, but sensing, your mind moving out into the world. Notice what it feels like to imagine your mind, not just in your head but all around you, in the world. As you breathe out, imagine the mind moving further and further out, sensing what is around you. If you are aware of sounds, let them be in your mind as well as in the world. While you are letting your mind move out, keep a sense of your body and the ground beneath you. Try to sit as if your awareness is balanced between what is inside you and what is outside.*

> *When it feels right, just let go of trying to do anything at all. Keep your posture and just relax so that you sit for a while without imposing any ideas on your experience. Let things be as they are.*

soul and spirit

I mentioned earlier that I would write more about the term 'spiritual'. My reservations about it are related to the way we experience ourselves in the world and how we use spiritual practice in relationship to our way through the world. James Hillman, in his essay 'On Soul and Spirit', writes, 'The spiritual point of view always posits itself as superior, and operates particularly well in a fantasy of transcendence among ultimates and absolutes.'[15]

It is worth reading the above quotation a few times. Typically, Hillman is being very challenging, and you might be inclined to pass over this with little thought, but I believe what Hillman is saying is very important. He is alluding to the tendency of people who consider themselves to be 'spiritual' to feel that they are in some sense above others and above the mundane world. This tendency to understand 'spiritual' practice as a concern with higher matters can cut us off from lived experience, and becomes a means of escape from, rather than engagement with, ourselves and the everyday world. On a collective level, it can lead to fanaticism; at worst, the belief that we are right and everyone else is wrong becomes the basis for evil actions such as persecution and all kinds of repression. On the level of the individual it can lead to what we might call a loss of 'soul'. Here, following Hillman, I am using the term 'soul' in a particular way. The word is sometimes used to refer to a part of us understood as somehow separate from our physical existence, an eternal part of us that will be liberated from the prison of the suffering body at death and, if we are lucky, will ascend to be with God. That is quite the opposite of what I mean. If you are a Billie Holiday fan, think of her singing 'Lover Man' and you will have some feeling for the sort of soul I am interested in. Singing is a particularly good metaphor because it is a deeply 'embodied' art. If you are a fine art fan, bring to mind a Rembrandt self-portrait. Or remember cooking a meal with care, fully devoting yourself to the cooking.

Soul, then, is not a thing; it is a quality that can be associated with an action or a particular thing. It is a quality that cannot be categorized or measured, cannot be rigidly defined. Nevertheless, it is the quality that gives our actions their depth and meaning. In meditation, it is the difference between meditating from the ego and meditating with the body, the difference between meditating to be in the world, and meditating as a means of transcending the world.

When we meditate from our heads or our egos, there is always an underlying anxiety, a grasping at experience, wanting something to happen. We have an idea imposed upon our felt experience. This cannot be completely avoided, we all do it. It can, however, be recognized and balanced by bringing the body, feeling, and sensations fully into awareness. It is a not possible to be aware of the body and to be lost in fantasy; when we are engaged with the body, fantasy has no room to proliferate.

'Soul', in the sense I am using the word, is also very much related to imagination, as opposed to fantasy. Here I mean fantasy as a attempt to feed the ego, such as fantasizing about winning a lottery, or an attractive person we have just met. By imagination I mean invoking an image that comes from somewhere deep inside us. It is not the product of our egos. This is why it has been traditionally associated with the muse, for it is as though it comes from somewhere else. Frustratingly, perhaps, the imagination, like soul, cannot be neatly defined, it is more a matter of feeling it. When we pay attention to the body, we open ourselves up to the imagination of soul, we open to the depths within us which might come into awareness as an image or a thought or just a feeling.

Hillman draws a helpful distinction between soul and spirit. He sees both as vital, but is keen to warn us of the dangers of spirit and spiritual practice without soul, although it is not possible to define precisely what he means here by soul, for one of soul's characteristics is that it is rather dark and indistinct, rather mysterious. Soul relates to the hidden parts of us, the bits that perhaps we would rather like to ignore, particularly if we see ourselves as spiritual aspirants. It makes itself known through dreams and those waking images and thoughts that are powerful but slip away when we try to grasp then. It is sensed on the edge of our awareness, like something seen out of the corner of the eye. In our story of the Buddha, we might say that in his time as an ascetic he lost touch with this vital aspect that I am calling soul. Soul is related to body, feelings, fantasy, fears, and decay. The would-be Buddha, as an ascetic, was trying to overcome the body, trying to release the spirit from the body, to separate spirit from soul. Spirit is dry and wants to ascend – it is related to light and fire – while soul is moist, to do with the earth, and tends towards descent. But each needs the other.

Later in the same essay, Hillman says,

> *We can experience soul and spirit interacting. At moments of intellectual concentration or transcendental meditation, soul invades with natural urges, memories, fantasies, and fears. At times of new psychological insights or experiences, spirit would quickly extract a meaning, put them into action, conceptualize them into rules. Soul sticks to the realm of experience and to reflections within experience. It moves indirectly in circular reasonings, where retreats are as important as advances, preferring labyrinths and corners, giving a metaphorical*

sense to life through such words as close, near, slow, and deep. Soul involves us in the pack and welter of phenomena and the flow of impressions. It is the 'patient' part of us. Soul is vulnerable and suffers; it is passive and remembers. It is water to the spirit's fire, like a mermaid who beckons the heroic spirit into the depths of passions to extinguish its certainty. Soul is imagination, a cavernous treasury – to use an image from St Augustine – a confusion and richness, both. Whereas spirit chooses the better part and seeks to make all one. Look up, says spirit, gain distance; there is something beyond and above, and what is above is always, and always superior.[16]

I hope that gives you a bit of a feeling for what I mean by soul, and why I am a little careful around the area of 'spiritual' practice. It is very easy for our meditation to take on the same texture as other activities in life, where we feel driven to 'do well'. We start to think in terms of having good or bad meditations. We experience our soul experiences as an intrusion into the clear bright place we think that meditation should be, a kind of white room free from the germs of our mind and body. This sort of idea arises when we think of meditation as being about just the spirit, about rising above the world. Of course, higher states do sometimes very clearly occur in meditation, and these can be very inspiring and important. We do not want to banish spirit. As long as these higher states are grounded in our real experience they are to be welcomed and enjoyed, but they should not become the sole aim of our practice. Soul keeps the spirit in the body; in terms of meditation it keeps the mind embodied, that is, in a sensational and feeling relationship with the body.

medtation: encouraging a sense of soul

Sit in your meditation posture. Become aware of your breath low in your body. You might try doing a cycle of abdominal breaths, particularly if you feel distracted. Just be aware of the ground beneath you. Do not force anything to happen but just gently encourage a sense of what it is like to sit on the earth. Softly imagine the earth as a living being, a living presence, as personified by the earth goddess. Don't try to make these thoughts too distinct, don't force then, just feel the earth supporting you. How does it feel to be supported by the earth? What is holding you from fully giving yourself to the ground, surrendering to being fully here, now.

Notice your distractions with kindness. Breathe into those thoughts. Don't try to get rid of them. Just let them, too, be supported by the ground. Use your breath to help you bring your awareness into your belly. Notice the sensations, the feelings, the emotions. Notice when the ego pulls away, notice if you try to impose ideas on the raw experience of being in your belly.

After a while, include the heart area. Notice what happens, any resistance to being in the heart. Notice the joy or the heartache. When the ego tries to appropriate the feeling of being in the belly and being in your heart, treat it with love. Tell yourself it is all right to feel what you feel. Notice your tendency to rationalize, argue, criticize. Notice when fantasies arise. See if you can feel the difference between fantasy that draws you away, and imagination that pulls you down into your heart, into your guts. All the time, remember the earth, supporting you without judgement, just as you are, in the wonder of your imperfections. Be like earth to yourself, without demand, just being with abiding, with what is there. Breathe into the grasping. When images or thoughts arise, do not judge them or try to make sense of them. Listen to them, let them speak for themselves. Do not think that this image must mean this or that, but see if you can just abide with your experience, with a sense of openness and care.

Keep gently returning to the ground and your body. Perhaps nothing much happens. Try to be all right with that. You cannot force soul; it will reveal itself in its own time. Be patient, and very gently encourage your awareness to be with your body, and any areas where you sense you hold on, that feel disconnected, or somehow negatively or positively charged. This could happen anywhere, but areas that correspond to the chakras are worth taking time to notice. Try noticing your throat, which often seems to be a place where we block energy and imagination from entering our awareness, where a split occurs between body and mind, heart and head, spirit and soul. Become aware of the base of your spine, the root chakra, notice the pelvic area including your genitals. Gently try to feel into the body, not just physically but also the quality of energy held in that particular area. Maintain a receptive attitude, a kind of attentive listening. Just as when you listen to music, certain feelings and emotions might arise, listen to the body and notice what arises. If a particular thought, image, or memory arises, just stay with it without elaborating on it. Just let it be there in your awareness without feeling that you have to interpret or interrogate it. Be attentive to your experience, but at the same time see if it is possible just to let it be. Before you finish, come back to your breath and fully relax. Then let go of the idea of doing anything at all. Just sit.

So the idea of soul and the idea of embodiment are related to each other, for by becoming increasingly embodied, becoming more aware of the sensational and feeling aspects of our everyday experience, we also invite an increased sense of soul into our lives. I find the idea of soulfulness very powerful in relation to our increasingly hectic and often superficial lives. Soul goes against the idea of progress in a linear sense. It circles and takes us backwards as well as forwards. To live soulfully means to have a sense of space and time in our lives, time for reflection, time to allow our experience to mature and deepen within us. It means that we do not fill up every minute of our waking lives. Perhaps the most important thing a meditation practice offers us is a space just to be.

Meditation offers us the space and time we need to come home to ourselves, and in this coming home we also come into a deeper relationship with soul, which is both the most intimate and the most universal aspect of ourselves. Over the page is a poem to end with, by William Carlos Williams, which captures a sense of both mindfulness and soul.

thursday

I have had my dream – like others –
and it has come to nothing, so that
I remain now carelessly
with feet planted on the ground
and look up at the sky –
feeling my clothes about me,
the weight of my body in my shoes,
the rim of my hat, air passing in and out
at my nose – and decide to dream no more.

notes

1 Ryokan, *One Robe, One Bowl*, John Stevens (trans.), Weatherhill 1977, p.33.

2 As told, for example, by Philip Kapleau in *The Three Pillars of Zen*, Doubleday 1989, pp.10–11.

3 The *Satipatthana Sutta* is the tenth sutta in the *Majjhima Nikaya*, or 'book of middle-length discourses'. This translation is by Soma Thera.

4 See Will Johnson's excellent book, *Aligned, Relaxed, Resilient* for a more detailed account of this approach to posture.

5 Quoted in James Hillman, *A Blue Fire*, HarperCollins, 1991.

6 As told, for example, in the *Mahasaccaka Sutta*, sutta 36 of the *Majjhima Nikaya*.

7 Gwendolyn Bays (trans.), *The Voice of the Buddha (Lalitavistara)*, Dharma Publishing 1983, pp.480–482.

8 As told, for example, by Mark Epstein in *Thoughts Without a Thinker*, Duckworth 1997.

9 This meditation is explained in full in the previous book in this series, *The Heart*, by Vessantara, Windhorse Publications 2006.

10 This is the story of Kisa Gotami, from the *Therigatha* or 'Poems of the Buddhist sisters', canto 10.

11 The *Angulimala Sutta*, the 86th sutta of the *Majjhima Nikaya*.

12 James Hillman, op.cit., p.201.

13 Quoted in Taitetsu Unno, *River of Fire, River of Water*, Doubleday 1998, p.50.

14 Richard Lewontin, 'The organism as the subject and object of evolution', *Scientia* 118:63–82, as quoted in Francisco J. Varela, *The Embodied Mind*, MIT Press 1993, p.198.

15 James Hillman, op.cit., p.121.

16 ibid., p.122.

The windhorse symbolizes the energy of the Enlightened mind carrying the truth of the Buddha's teachings to all corners of the world. On its back the windhorse bears three jewels: a brilliant gold jewel represents the Buddha, the ideal of Enlightenment, a sparkling blue jewel represents the teachings of the Buddha, the Dharma, and a glowing red jewel, the community of the Buddha's enlightened followers, the Sangha. Windhorse Publications, through the medium of books, similarly takes these three jewels out to the world.

Windhorse Publications is a Buddhist publishing house, staffed by practising Buddhists. We place great emphasis on producing books of high quality, accessible and relevant to those interested in Buddhism at whatever level. Drawing on the whole range of the Buddhist tradition, our books include translations of traditional texts, commentaries, books that make links with Western culture and ways of life, biographies of Buddhists, and works on meditation.

As a charitable institution we welcome donations to help us continue our work. We also welcome manuscripts on aspects of Buddhism or meditation. For orders and catalogues log on to www.windhorsepublications.com or contact:

Windhorse Publications	Perseus Distribution	Windhorse Books
11 Park Road	1094 Flex Drive	P O Box 574
Birmingham	Jackson, TN 38301	Newtown NSW 2042
B13 8AB	USA	Australia
UK		

Windhorse Publications is an arm of the Friends of the Western Buddhist Order, which has more than sixty centres on four continents. Through these centres, members of the Western Buddhist Order offer regular programmes of events for the general public and for more experienced students. These include meditation classes, public talks, study on Buddhist themes and texts, and bodywork classes such as t'ai chi, yoga, and massage. The FWBO also runs several retreat centres and the Karuna Trust, a fundraising charity that supports social welfare projects in the slums and villages of India.

Many FWBO centres have residential spiritual communities and ethical businesses associated with them. Arts activities are encouraged too, as is the development of strong bonds of friendship between people who share the same ideals. In this way the FWBO is developing a unique approach to Buddhism, not simply as a set of techniques, but as a creatively directed way of life for people living in the modern world.

If you would like more information about the FWBO please visit the website at www.fwbo.org or write to:

London Buddhist Centre	Aryaloka	Sydney Buddhist Centre
51 Roman Road	14 Heartwood Circle	24 Enmore Road
London	Newmarket NH 03857	Sydney NSW 2042
E2 0HU	USA	Australia
UK		

ALSO FROM WINDHORSE PUBLICATIONS

CHANGE YOUR MIND:
A PRACTICAL GUIDE TO BUDDHIST MEDITATION

PARAMANANDA

Buddhism is based on the truth that, with effort, we can change the way we are. But how? Among the many methods Buddhism has to offer, meditation is the most direct. It is the art of getting to know one's own mind and learning to encourage what is best in us.

This bestseller is an approachable and thorough guide to meditation, based on traditional material but written in a light and modern style. Colourfully illustrated with anecdotes and tips from the author's experience as a meditator and teacher, it also offers refreshing inspiration to seasoned meditators.

208 pages, with photographs
ISBN 1 899579 75 3
£9.99/$13.95/€13.95

Inspiring, calming, and friendly, this book makes the exercises and meditation techniques ... easy to follow through.... If you've always thought meditation might be a good idea, by found other step-by-step guides lacking in spirit, this book could finally get you going.
Here's Health

A DEEPER BEAUTY:
BUDDHIST REFLECTIONS ON EVERYDAY LIFE

PARAMANANDA

In *A Deeper Beauty*, Paramananda speaks directly to our hearts about what is truly important to us, whether we are making a cup of tea or sitting at the bedside of a dying friend. Using simple exercises, reflections, and meditations, we can awaken to the magic of being fully present in each moment.

Paramananda draws on his experience as a hospice worker and his many years as a Buddhist meditation teacher in an imaginative and down-to-earth way. He offers us courage, kindness, and joy in our search for meaning.

We are invited to a deeper intimacy with ourselves and the world – to plunge beneath the surface of our ordinary lives to find a deeper beauty.

208 pages
ISBN 1 899579 44 3
£8.99/$16.95/€16.95

ALSO IN THIS SERIES

THE BREATH

VESSANTARA

The breath: always with us, necessary to our very existence, but often unnoticed. Yet giving it attention can transform our lives.

This is a very useful combination of practical instruction on the mindfulness of breathing with much broader lessons on where the breath can lead us. Vessantara, a meditator of many years experience, offers us:

> * Clear instruction on how to meditate on the breath
> * Practical ways to integrate meditation into our lives
> * Suggestions for deepening calm and concentration
> * Advice on how to let go and dive into experience
> * Insights into the lessons of the breath

The Breath returns us again and again to the fundamental and precious experience of being alive.

144 pages
ISBN 1 899579 69 9
£6.99/$10.95/€10.95

An interesting in-depth investigation into the art of breathing.
Yoga magazine